THE

SUSTAINABLE

Y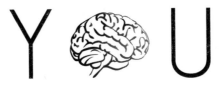U

THE
SUSTAINABLE
Y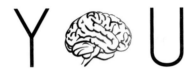U

SOMATICS
AND THE
MYTH OF AGING

THE SMART WAY
TO ACHIEVE AND
MAINTAIN YOUR
BEST BODY

JOHN LOUPOS, H.S.E., M.S.

LANGDON STREET PRESS   MINNEAPOLIS

Langdon Street Press
212 3rd Avenue North, Suite 290
Minneapolis, MN 55401
612.455.2293
www.langdonstreetpress.com

ISBN: 978-1-936782-13-0
LCCN: 2011925903

Distributed by Itasca Books

Printed in the United States of America

PLEASE NOTE

This book is intended to familiarize readers with the theories, principles, and efficacy of somatic education. It is not meant to train readers in the application of its technique for use on others. The information herein is not intended to diagnose, treat, cure, or prevent any disease. All information relating to medical conditions, health issues, products, and treatments are not meant as a substitute for the advice of your physician or other medical professional. The author offers guidance on several movement patterns that readers are invited to experiment with, but only if there are no contraindications to doing so. Consult with your physician or medical professional before making changes to medications or doctor recommended programs of any kind.

John Loupos is certified as a Hanna somatic educator (HSE) and as a clinical somatic educator (CSE). Though both certifications represent functionally similar brands, Hanna Somatic Education is the longer-standing term. This term or its more casual abbreviated derivatives (somatic education, somatics, or HSE) are used throughout this book. In each case the reference is the same. Appropriate resources for training in somatics, and for locating a qualified practitioner, are listed in Chapter 17, Final Words: Resources—Where to Go from Here.

CONTENTS

PART 1: GENERAL THEORIES OF SOMATICS / 1

PART 2: APPLIED SOMATICS / 83

PART 3: MUSINGS, ESSAYS, QUESTIONS, AND ANSWERS / 143

PART 4: SOMATIC MOVEMENT PATTERNS / 203

FOREWORD

In some ways, John Loupos and I could not be more different. He is a Tai Chi and martial arts expert, and expert in Thomas Hanna's practice of Somatics. I am a biological psychiatrist, an expert in sociobiology, and a reductionist. He is an expert in Qi (pronounced *chee*), the Chinese concept of life energy. I am an expert in psychopharmacology, the use of medications for mental disorders. Theoretically, we are as different as different could be.

But we find common ground in a firm belief in human free will and potential. John Loupos' new book, *The Sustainable You* outlines the theory and practice of Hanna Somatics, which is, as I understand it, a practice of expanding the use of the human brain to improve communication with muscles and the rest of the body, resulting in vastly improved levels of function and pain reduction. The actual treatments by somatics practitioners take, in most cases, just a few sessions and claim dramatic improvements for people with back pain, strokes, muscle contractures, and even sexual dysfunction. These clinical sessions work best when coupled with the daily practice of exercises that although painless are far from simple, because they involve teaching the brain to overcome "sensorimotor amnesia" in order to reconnect incoming signals to the brain with outgoing improvement in striated muscle responsiveness. Many of these uniquely designed exercises entail painstaking detail in awareness and then control. The book includes discussion of the theory of

Somatics, case histories, and a sampler of exercises to be done at home, daily.

I hurt. I just had a knee replacement and was told that even with extensive conventional physical therapy I have an extension contracture of my new knee, and it will never get better. How I wish that I could fly to Boston to meet John Loupos and have him attend to my poor knee. Conventional medicine has given up, as happens so often. Somatics offers hope where conventional medicine has failed. I like this book because the neurophysiology is correct and sophisticated. It is not "New Age" hocus-pocus. I understand, as a scientist, how improved proprioception and afferent neuronal function plus consciousness should result in improved efferent signaling and neuromuscular function. Learning to control the muscles of the perineum, for example, should be similar to learning to play the piano—awareness, practice, then improved control and finally improved habits of control. I especially like John Loupos's lack of shyness dealing with the urogenital system, including sexuality.

Given the limitations of modern allopathic medicine, the prohibitive costs of treatments, and the side effects of invasive procedures, the world needs more information, realistic and informed alternatives, about ways to feel good and improve health into old age. I am looking forward to trying the exercises myself, and committing to using this method as a step in my own recovery from knee surgery. The only people who would not benefit from reading this book are those who want to be passive, who want other people to take care of them, and who don't really want to work towards better health. For anyone else with chronic pain or disability, read this book.

-Judith Eve Lipton, M.D.
Distinguished Fellow of the American Psychiatric Association,
clinical faculty, University of Washington, author of *The Myth of Monogamy: Fidelity and Infidelity in Animals and People* (2001) and *Payback! Why we retaliate, redirect aggression, and seek revenge* (2011)

FOREWORD

I first met John Loupos at the 30th Annual Zhang Sanfeng (Tai Chi) Festival in East Stroudsburg, Pennsylvania, where we were fellow vendors of books and CDs. I was suffering from bursitis in my right shoulder, which had abated but was not completely healed. A budding somatics practitioner, John was itching to get his hands on my shoulder; and I was more than willing to have him practice on me. So I had my first somatics experience in the back corner of the conference sales room with a more substantial follow-up later.

Needless to say, it worked wonders and I became an instant enthusiastic convert, purchasing the *Somatics* book and *The Myth of Aging* CD series, both by Thomas Hanna. Practicing at home, I loved Thomas Hanna's style and was also thrilled by the physical gentleness and mental challenge of the exercises. I soon converted my husband, and we have used somatics ever since, although (and as John points out in the book) typically—not consistently and regularly, but rather as physical tension made it a necessity.

Since that summer of 2005, I have seen John several times, notably as patient in his Cohasset studio/clinic, and stayed in contact via email after moving to other parts of the country. Continuing my own work on the exploration of Daoist modes of self-cultivation and working on the history of qigong and Taijiquan (Chinese healing exercises), I have had ample opportunity to use somatics theory and experience to explain how and why certain traditional Daoist moves work and produce the benefits they claim. Overall, somatics has been very good to me, both personally and professionally, not to mention in my marriage; since somatics happily cleared up my husband's persistent long-term back pain.

I am deeply honored to write a foreword for John's wonderful new book, *The Sustainable You: Somatics and the Myth of Aging*. Reading through it inspired me to jump-start our somatics practice yet again, and finally—after purchasing them five years ago—to work through all the other Thomas Hanna guided media that deal more specifically with wrists, shoulders, neck, back, and hips. I am eager to try John's new routines described here, especially for shoulders and lower abdomen. And I am resolved to continue my practice—this time without interruption, making healthy stretches a daily priority and not an "as needed" convenience.

John's book adds a valuable and greatly appreciated dimension to our understanding and practice of somatics. He gives a thoroughly researched and clearly presented overview of the practice, including overall theory, scientific underpinnings, detailed protocols, connection to Taijiquan and martial arts, as well as the social and political relevance of somatics. Without repeating or taking away from Hanna's original volume, John brings our appreciation of the practice to a new level, exploring it from numerous angles and creating a new venue of understanding that will help practitioners deepen their experience, and newcomers discover this amazing method of self-healing.

-Livia Kohn, Ph.D.
Professor Emerita, Religion and East Asian Studies at Boston University, and executive editor of *Journal of Daoist Studies*. Dr. Kohn has practiced Taijiquan, qigong, meditation, and yoga for over twenty years and has written or edited more than 25 books on these subjects. www.liviakohn.com

ACKNOWLEDGMENTS

Many thanks are in order to the following individuals for their help and support in bringing this text to fruition. First, I extend my thanks to the late Thomas Hanna Ph.D. for his courage and conviction, and for his vision in pioneering modern somatics. I am also indebted to my trainers at the Somatics Systems Institute in Northampton, Massachusetts: Steve Aronstein, Karen Hewitt, Pam Bladine, and Marilyn Warnock. Each of these fine teachers lent their encouragement, support, and endorsement while I endeavored to capture in so many words a brief synopsis of their many decades of service as somatic trainers and educators. Marilyn, in particular, was meticulous in reviewing and offering helpful suggestions for my manuscript in its early stages. Special thanks go to my longtime partner, Christina, for her patience and support while my manuscript developed. Thanks to Tim Comrie at YMAA Publications for his help with key graphics, and to Clayton Handleman for photography. Thanks are due as well to my Tai Chi students, Bill Stenson M.D., Steve Golden, M.D., Mark Kremen M.D., and Joanne Kornoelje, and also to Mitchell Fleisher M.D., and Bradford C. Bennett Ph.D. for reviewing and extending their learned opinions on this text during its development. I am indebted to Judith Lipton, M.D. for her foreword, as I am to Livia Kohn Ph.D. for her helpful suggestions, and for her foreword.

I am very grateful to my somatics colleagues who were sufficiently enthused about the prospects for this book to share from their case files in support of this project. These include Martha Peterson, Jon Aronstein, Karen Hewitt, Katherine Kerber, Jonathan Hunt, Lawrence Gold, Steve Aronstein, and Laura Gates, who also contributed several drawings. Thanks to Karin Scholz Grace for sharing her perspective on HSE and yoga. I am particularly indebted to Eleanor Criswell-Hanna for her careful review and helpful suggestions, and deeply grateful for her personal seal of approval on this body of work. My editor, Marly Cornell, provided invaluable service and was fun to work with. Finally, I would hardly have any basis for writing from experience if not for the many clients I've been privileged to work with over the years.

PREFACE

I was a child of the sixties. That, along with my being a veteran of more than forty-five years at martial arts, during which I've specialized at Tai Chi and qigong (chi kung), and having a clinical background in classical homeopathy, and considering that I'm an organic gardening enthusiast and fitness buff, I have always regarded myself as highly attuned to healthy living. For many decades I have been a proponent of self-reliance and taking responsibility for my own well-being, ascribing to an approach probably best described as "proactive preventative natural healthcare." Commensurate with this line of thinking I regularly sought out deep tissue massage, chiropractic and applied kinesiology sessions, nutritional consultation, and, occasionally, acupuncture, opting for conventional medicine and pharmacology only when absolutely necessary. However, as the years and decades began to exact their toll, I observed that these therapeutic, albeit more natural, modalities came to seem less an elective indulgence on my part and increasingly more a necessity in keeping at bay the debilitative effects of aging on my body. It wasn't until my preferred non-conventional therapeutic modalities failed to provide effective reprieve from a lingering shoulder injury that the thought first occurred to me: *Yes, I do all these good things for myself; but, no, they were not seeming effective as long-term solutions for my own optimal health.*

I didn't want to be stuck in dependence on my chosen natural health and wellness resources any more than I wanted to be stuck on the conventional medical system. There had to be a more effective way to maintain my health and wellness while avoiding the revolving door syndrome that so often characterizes healthcare, regardless of one's therapeutic ethic.

The same shoulder injury led me to discover Hanna Somatic Education, the subject of this book. I found in this method the means of resolving, as opposed to merely holding in abeyance, the whole checklist of neuromuscular problems—aches, pains, stiffness, and spasms—that had been plaguing my body for some time. Prior to somatics those issues portended a trajectory of physical decline, all my various healthy body resources notwithstanding. With somatics in my life, I'm no longer stuck in the "therapy/temporary improvement/relapse/more therapy" cycle. Instead, I find myself able to provide for my body in a manner that is perfectly adequate to my health and wellness needs. I simply set aside ten–thirty minutes each day for practicing somatic movement patterns. This is all the time it takes to remind the cortical self-sensing aspects of my brain how to maintain a differentiated overview of the potential problem areas in my body. My practice of somatics has effectively replaced my previous reliance on other health modalities, saving me time, money, and untold aggravation. Somatics is easy, effective, quick, and fun. And, having once learned this method, it costs me nothing whatsoever to apply these skills whenever and wherever I feel the need.

I often meet other people who are stuck in their own revolving door, prompting me to reflect, *if only these people had some awareness of somatics, they might be better able to assume fuller charge of their own lives and well-being, just as I have.* This book is for all those people who would like to assume fuller charge of their own well-being and dispense once and for all with their own revolving doors.

INTRODUCTION

"Before I die I want to see enough change happening...to say
I've helped things along a bit...What's the point of living if
I don't leave something for others? I've got certain talents,
certain understandings; it's in some sense my own personal
obligation to myself and other human beings to help them
in any way I can. It has nothing to do with power. It has to
do with loving other people and being concerned with the
human condition."[1]
~Thomas Hanna Ph.D. (1928–90)

The sentiment expressed above typified the late Thomas Hanna, Ph.D. Hanna made every effort to leave the world a better place for his time in it. The health and wellness methods (referred to herein as "somatics") that were developed by Hanna are based on those "certain talents and understandings," and collectively represent an approach that is unique to the human condition. Countless other modalities purport to ease common neuromuscular maladies, from mild discomforts to outright pain; but results often vary widely between patients, and depending on their circumstances. Quite often persons seeking relief end up with temporary relief at best (palliation), instead of "problem solved."

No other conventional or non-conventional healing method approaches the elimination of pain and the restoration of overall personal health in the manner of somatics. Though other modalities may eliminate or ease pain and

---

1 *East West* interview with Mirka Knaster, 2/89.

suffering in some cases, somatics is often effective where other methods are not. Therefore, it is my great pleasure to share with readers the philosophical, theoretical, practical, and technical aspects of modern somatics.

Though I only entered this field some thirteen years after Hanna's passing, I have been passionate about somatic education since my first hands-on encounter. I came to somatics with an injury that had me in constant discomfort and occasional outright pain, with a much restricted range of motion. I developed what is known in the vernacular as a "frozen" shoulder. Being a martial arts professional, this injury went beyond mere inconvenience. My career was at risk. I pursued a litany of alternative approaches, including chiropractic, applied kinesiology, deep tissue massage, homeopathy, acupuncture, and even more conventional physical therapy to resolve my shoulder issue, all to no avail. Serendipitously, I came across Thomas Hanna's book, *Somatics*, which led me to the Somatic Systems Institute in Northampton, Massachusetts. A single one-hour session there was all that was required to put my shoulder right, restored to a hundred percent working order after a year of constant pain and stiffness. It seemed a bit surreal. It was too easy.

Amidst my delight and amazement at having recovered full use of my shoulder in such short order, the implications for me and my students were immediately obvious. I inquired about professional training and signed on for the first available practitioner training module. Since early in my training I've been fortunate to help many other people in similar dire need. My only regret is having missed the opportunity to meet Thomas Hanna who, by my way of thinking, was one of the great unheralded minds of modern times.

I undertook the task of writing this book about somatic education, hoping to make an important addition to the field. Thomas Hanna already wrote what I, and many other somatics professionals, regard as the definitive book on somatic education. As many times as I've read *Somatics*, I still find myself musing on how, or even if, it might be possible to improve on his original work, so thorough and articulate was the original text. Even so, I remain committed, along with a host of others, to ensuring that Hanna's legacy, in the form of qualified practitioners utilizing his methods, is propagated in order to lessen unnecessary human pain and suffering.

My intent, therefore, is not to improve on Hanna's original work so much as to complement it by offering an expanded perspective on his legacy. This undertaking seems to me especially timely given the current dual concerns over our already overburdened healthcare system, coupled with the growing numbers of aging baby boomers advancing through their middle years and beyond toward that stage of life when the culmination of a life lived is most likely to exact its heaviest toll. In the pages that follow I shall present an argument for how somatic education can provide some measure of relief, both for individuals and for our healthcare system overall.

Since the time of René Descartes,[2] conventional Western science, technology, and medicine have been largely defined by an approach that is best described as reductionist and mechanistic. According to this approach everything is held to be assembled at some level by basic building blocks, and by the assumption that these units can be dismantled and reduced to their smallest denominators, their secrets revealed, and then reassembled intact, in many cases for gainful pursuit. This approach has many claims to its efficacy, and rightfully so. Were it not for advances made in the name of Western science and medicine I might be writing with charcoal on papyrus instead of typing away on my computer. Though hubris and shortsightedness have, at times, reflected poorly on conventional science and medicine, we have a great deal to be thankful for in this Western model. Advances in science and technology characterize and define modern life.

It may therefore strike proponents of this model as somewhat heretical to suggest that any promise of powerful healing, and even optimal wellness, exists beyond its mechanical and reductionist borders. Granted, for individuals already accustomed to nontraditional therapeutic modalities, e.g, traditional Chinese medicine (TCM), classical homeopathy, ayurvedic medicine, and assorted indigenous systems, such a claim as this proffers no great revela-

---

2 René Descartes 1596–1650.

tion. Even so, the special promise of this book is to familiarize readers with a revolutionary method of healing and wellness that is founded in conventional neurophysiology, but which calls for no technical, mechanical, or intrusive therapeutic measures. Rather, simple education is the means by which life-changing gains may be achieved by implementing the user-friendly methods described throughout this text.

The last hundred or so years have shown us mind-boggling advances on many fronts, from the smallest of the small to the largest and farthest imaginable. Scientific, technical, and medical marvels aside, the twentieth century was also characterized by certain, more individually relevant though less-widely touted, advances. These advances are credited to a small field of somatic innovators, each of whom struggled against prevailing wisdom in seeking acceptance for his or her theories and methods.[3] The most recent of these was Thomas Hanna, Ph.D.

Hanna was an early protégé and colleague of Moshe Feldenkrais, the founder of Functional Integration and Awareness Through Movement. Hanna's approach differed from that of Feldenkrais and other somatic predecessors in that Hanna borrowed from conventional science and medicine to add in 1) a comprehensive diagnostic theory, 2) a general somatic theory of sensorimotor process, and 3) a method of somatic education that engaged the learner's motor actions to involve the full capacity of the sensorimotor feedback loop.

Hanna's somatic education system strikes me as particularly unique in that it sprang from a philosophical as well as practical mandate held by its founder. Thomas Hanna saw himself as a pragmatist because of his belief that human beings have the wherewithal to solve problems, both extrinsically (via science, technology, and the like), and intrinsically within their own bodies,

---

3   Among these notables are F. Mathias Alexander, Elsa Gindler, and Gerda Alexander.

or somas.[4,5] Hanna's great passion was in facilitating optimal wellness and total harmony between body and consciousness so that mankind might learn to live freely and painlessly with an enhanced ability for self-determination.

In the years before his death Thomas Hanna conducted a series of seminars to introduce his new educational method to the public. His weekend trainings in guided movement regularly drew hundreds of people. He was a prolific teacher and writer, yet he was not able to see his dream of truly wide-scale propagation of his teaching method fully realized before his untimely passing, at least not on any scale that extended considerably beyond the scope of his own practice. Happily, Hanna did plant the seeds of his accomplishments, making it possible for others to pick up where he left off.

Approximately parallel to Hanna's work, and in the years since his death, there have been impressive advances in the neurosciences. These sciences have evolved on a vastly more comprehensive (and well-funded) scale as compared to homespun somatic disciplines. "Neuroscience" is an umbrella term for many evolving subfields, e.g., neuropsychology, psychoneuroimmunology, etc. New branches and applications of neuroscience are still being unveiled— neuroeconomics, neuroforensics, neurotheology, neuroaesthetics, and neuro- ethics, to name a few.

Throughout this book I cite the work and accomplishments of many leading brain researchers, men and women whose cutting-edge research offers invaluable insight into the deepest workings of the brain and nervous system, including the brain's potential for neuroplasticity (adaptive change). Much of what is revealed as a result of research on the brain has direct relevance to somatics. With respect to the various sciences, I want to be clear from the start that this is a book primarily about sensorimotor health and wellness. This is about getting your muscles and your brain to collaborate optimally as regards

---

4   "Somatology: An Introduction to Somatic Philosophy and Psychology," Pt 1, *Somatics Journal*, XV, 2, 07.
5   In his teachings Hanna used the term "soma" rather than "body" to denote the individual person or being from the individual's own first-person perspective. Throughout this text I have deliberately opted for the more colloquial term "body" to keep things simple, even though HSE addresses aspects of the whole person.

voluntary motor function, so that you can learn to live in your own body in the best way possible. This information is for and about you.

As fascinating as the various neurosciences are on their merits, the upshot is that conventional brain research has not, to date, offered the majority of people who fall well within the mean any prospect of rapid non-pharmacological relief from ordinary bodily pain. No brain-related academic or medical research has revealed the cause or delivered a cure for common back pain, or for the debilitating effects of aging on the body. Somatics, on the other hand, has effectively done just that, perhaps not for all of the pain of all people all of the time, but certainly in a way and to an extent that should inspire health providers and lay people everywhere to sit up and take notice. Somatics has exposed the "myth of aging" for what it is.

As a pioneer in the field of somatic health and wellness, Thomas Hanna left more than his fair share on the table to upgrade the human condition. The seeds he sowed have slowly taken root, and the educational and wellness methods he developed are now on the brink of full flourish.

PART I

GENERAL THEORIES OF SOMATICS

I sat in my office, having just returned the prior evening from my first weekend of training as a future Hanna somatic educator. My classmates and I spent the previous four days absorbing lectures on somatics theory. Among the various tidbits I committed to memory were words of assurance offered by one of my instructors—that this somatics method works so well that even in the event that we plied our skills inexpertly we might still see dramatic improvement. Along with theory, our class was introduced during this inaugural weekend to the basic technique of "assisted pandiculation" (using gentle touch and pressure maneuvers to provide feedback to, and generate arousal at, the voluntary cortex as a means of addressing chronic muscle tension) though we were not schooled in pandicular application in the context of formal somatics protocols.

My phone rang. There, on the other end, was my first ever client, explaining how she'd had a stroke, and that her stroke-side hand had been bound up in a tight fist ever since. Could I help her?

"Can you come right over?" Thirty minutes later I was aghast as I peered out my window to observe two assistants lowering this woman from her car into a wheelchair, her stroke-damaged left side all a'twitch. *Was I in over my head?* We chatted for a short bit and I made it clear that I could make no promises regarding her condition. Then I undertook to apply my newly acquired skills in pandiculating her bound-up fist. Within five minutes, and for the first time since her stroke some three years earlier, her fist opened easily and completely, and the tears rolled down her face.

Geesh, I thought, *this stuff really works!*

CHAPTER 1

WHAT IS THE MYTH OF AGING?

"The great enemy of the truth is very often not the lie—
deliberate, contrived, and dishonest—but the myth, persistent, persuasive, and unrealistic. Belief in myths allows the
comfort of opinion without the discomfort of thought."
~John F. Kennedy

What is Aging?

Before we jump feet first into myth-busting, please note that the subtitle of
this book refers to "the myth of aging," and not "the aging myth," or "aging
is a myth." Aging is *not* a myth. Aging is very real, and I don't discount for a
moment that aging, as such, is an inescapable fact of life. Yet there are certain
popularly held misconceptions about aging; and I have set about herein to
expose perhaps the most insidious myth of all—that as we get older we must
also experience the decline of aging in preordained ways. First, though, I
think some brief attention to what aging is—and is not—is in order.

It doesn't take a brain scientist to know that aging means getting older.
Aging is something that everybody can relate to because we all age, and
because there are certain *de facto* truths surrounding the myth. Beyond the
given—that aging does mean *getting older*—we actually may require the services of a brain scientist, and other scientists as well, to determine what it
means to "age." Many scientists (in many scientific fields) are not in clear
agreement as to what, exactly, the aging process necessarily entails. One rea-

son for this absence of consensus is that people age *differently*. Another reason is that not all parts of the body age at the same pace, or in the same way.

Perhaps the most important reason of all is that much of what is entailed with the aging process is subjective, meaning that to some degree at least, we are just as young or as old as we feel ourselves to be. Some people are old at fifty, while others are still young at seventy-five. Much of the pain and stiffness, as well as loss of ease and agility, that people experience as they get older is idiopathic, meaning it is due to an unspecified origin or cause. Finally, many of those learned minds committed to exploring the phenomenon of human aging do so through the tinted lens of their particular persuasion.

Brain scientists look for a neural basis to explain the markers of aging, geneticists for family histories and genetic dispositions. Biogerentologists and nutritionists may see chemical imbalance or too many free radicals stemming from diet, while sociologists explore for usefulness and social meaning. Microbiologists may presuppose a genetic clock as determined by a finite numbers of cell divisions.[1] Psychologists may be concerned with the effect on the mind, subjectively or objectively, of maturation in the context of growing older. All the while, your family doctor has you watching your cholesterol and blood pressure. What many of us already know firsthand, and without a doubt, are the ever-narrowing limits imposed on our bodies by the process of growing older. What all these scientists are supposed to have in common is that they take a scientific approach in which a full range of possibilities are explored prior to arriving at conclusions (at least in theory).

Stemming from my interest in somatic education, I have a vested interest in the neurophysiology of the aging brain, because so much of what happens with the body can be traced to the brain. In reading much of what has been written about the brain by leading figures in this field, I found myself struck frankly by the absence of information, or even perspectives, addressing in any substantive fashion the connections between aging brains and the neuromuscular aspects of aging bodies. We see ample attention paid to rare

---

1 Known as the Hayflick limit.

but newsworthy degenerative "conditions" that occasionally garner attention in the media, and also to commonly recognized neuropathologies such as Alzheimer's and Parkinson's diseases, as well as traumatic events like strokes. Yet little of what I've read even ventured the possibility that there might be more than a casual connection between the physical decline associated with normal everyday aging and the willful brain, or that at least some of the physiological effects of aging might be subject to the brain's voluntary review.

This book is primarily designed to teach you how to live in your body in the best and most sustainable way. One effect of learning to live in your body in the best way, with somatics, is the understanding that much of the neuromuscular decline normally attributed to aging can be mitigated. Notably, this benefit is applicable regardless of chronological age. Somatics is not just for older persons wishing to stave off the effects of aging. Somatics is for *any*one who finds the prospect of enhanced neuromuscular intelligence, and the ability to more live freely in your body, as an appealing scenario.

The Myth

Thomas Hanna, in a stroke of genius, nicknamed his core set of movement patterns *The Myth of Aging* series.[2] More than some offhand catch phrase, this label begs a bit of scrutiny as it underscores the very nature of Hanna's Somatic Education. A myth is a belief or set of beliefs, often unproven or false, that has accrued around a person, an institution, or a phenomenon, and upon which other beliefs or values may be based. History, even to the present day, is rife with examples of broad-stroke social belief systems premised

---

2 In addition to the eight movement patterns comprising *The Myth of Aging* series, Thomas Hanna composed ten other sets of movement patterns, each containing a series of six–eight sequential lessons arranged according to body areas or bodily conditions. See Resources in Chapter 17 to learn more.

solely on myth.[3] Thomas Hanna saw the currently held beliefs about aging, specifically our collective assumptions about certain of the "inevitabilities" presumed to accompany the aging process, as just exactly that—a myth. In fact, our aging myth has roots dating all the way back to ancient Greece when the fabled Sphinx queried Oedipus thus, "What walks on four legs in the morning, two legs in the afternoon, and three legs in the evening?" The answer of course is man, as per the presumptive decline that necessarily accompanies the aging process, mandating the use of a cane in one's later years.

The particular myth debunked by Hanna is this: As people grow older their bodies inevitably decline along a downward trajectory, usually from middle age onward. This decline is known to be inevitable because it happens to the great majority of people as they age and move steadily toward death. Because this decline happens to so many people, it is the norm. Because it is the norm, it is "normal." Therefore, this decline is what each of us must necessarily expect our own future to hold.

Herein we have the myth upon which society's expectations are based. However, the logic of this myth is skewed; and, further, it is decidedly unscientific. Yet, this myth seems to carry with it the full weight and sanction of Western science and medicine for no other reason than the seeming truism that people's bodies do decline as they get older. Unimaginable sums of money have been invested in both a mindset and a social infrastructure, all premised on the supposed validity of the aging myth. Modern conventional science and medicine have hardly a clue that the steady trajectory of human decline, with much of the pain and suffering sadly concomitant to it is, in fact, not inevitable, at least not in a qualitative sense. Much of the attrition and many of the degenerative effects normally attributed to the aging process are avoidable and even reversible.

---

3 Examples of such popular or scientific/medical myths can be seen in but a small sampling: 1) Earth is the center of the universe around which all other celestial bodies orbit. 2) Cigarette smoking does not pose a health hazard (as recently as the 1980s). 3) Modern pharmaceutical medicine will eradicate disease by the 21st century. 4) We're born with all the neurons we will ever have, those being incapable of repair or regeneration. All these myths have been debunked.

The degenerative aspects of the aging process, at least as regards neuromuscular decline (imbalance, pain, stiffness, etc.),
stem from little more than the effects of an *archeology of insults*
against the body. The cumulative effect of these insults—in incrementally resetting the brain's default mode for motor behavior to a
progressively lower standard of performance and response—provides the basis for the aging myth.

Of course, common sense dictates that there's no stopping the chronol-
ogy of aging. The hours, the days, and the years march on by, no matter
what we do: we're born; we live, and in the end we all die. But the qualitative
aspects of how we live our lives and find ourselves impacted by events that
occur as we age are unquestionably much more within our realm of control
than conventional wisdom would have us believe.

Somatics may or may not have an effect on human longevity, in terms
of life extension. Life extension, however, is not our goal. What we seek to
achieve is a quality of life or, to borrow a concept from Dr. Andrew Weil,
a "compression of morbidity."[4] Somatics can help us manage the trajectory
of neuromuscular decline as we age to insure that we retain a greater ease
and freedom about the body for a longer time than might otherwise be the
case by minimizing the effects of insults. Much of the recent research on
aging has focused on preservation of mental faculties. An alternate view is
presented in the words of John Ratey, M.D., clinical associate professor of
psychiatry at Harvard Medical School: "...a sound mind won't do you much
good if your body fails."[5]

The important premise to grasp is the spectrum of cumulative effects
that stem from this archeology of alleged insults. The problem, for most peo-

---

4 Andrew Weil, M.D., *Healthy Aging: A Lifelong Guide to Your Physical and Spiritual Well-
Being*. Knopf, 2005.
5 John J. Ratey, M.D., *Spark: The Revolutionary New Science of Exercise and the Brain*.
Little Brown, 2008.

ple, derives from layer upon layer of insults incurred over a lifetime of living.

So, what exactly is an "insult?" An insult may be thought of as any experience, real or imagined, that (dis)stresses or "offends" the organism. That's YOU, your body and your mind.[6] Within somatics, our concern is confined to the effects of these insults on the functioning of the sensorimotor/ neuromuscular system. Regarding such insults, we can gain some better appreciation of their impact by assigning them, more or less arbitrarily, to one of three levels that I have contrived for ease of understanding.

First, though, a bit of a primer, so you can have a basis for understanding how insults affect the body as they do. The body's design is somewhat analogous to a car in that it has many different parts and systems, most of which are organized around a central frame. While a car's frame is made of rigid steel, the body's frame is made up of movable skeletal components—bones. These bones have no sentient value, meaning they cannot think to act in any way on their own. Bones only move when muscles make them move. The voluntary muscles of the motor system also have no will of their own. Muscles only act at the pleasure of the brain; and, when the muscles act, they do one thing, and one thing only—they contract. This begs the question: How is it that muscles know to contract or not contract? Muscular performance hinges on a seamless communication system between muscles and brain, a communication that occurs via sensory and motor (sensorimotor) nerve pathways. This communication network is delicate, and easily compromised by insults of various types. Insults can result in muscles becoming "stuck" in various degrees of contraction, also known as hypertonus. Significantly, not all insults have the same degree of effect on your body's muscles. We can gain some better appreciation of the effects of various insults by assigning them, more or less arbitrarily, to one of three levels which I have contrived for ease of understanding. Let's take a closer look as these different levels.

---

6 See Chapter 9, "Insults: How They Occur and How Their Effects Accumulate."

Insult Upon Insult

The first level involves "minor" insults, which are often benign issues that hardly command or even warrant attention. Examples of "first level" insults might include slumping while you watch television (or read this book), an emotionally stressful day at work or school, or a sub-optimally nutritious meal. Other possible entries to this list could include a night of restless sleep, pushing yourself when overtired, always carrying a handbag or book bag over the same shoulder or a wallet always tucked into the same back pocket, parents toting young children about on their hips, or any of a litany of other low-magnitude experiences falling into the very unscientific category of simply "not being good for you."

These are just samplings of simple direct-cause insults, not even taking into account secondary insults from primary causes, such as when the stress of commuting to work in heavy traffic causes a stiff neck that results in a headache and acute shoulder pain. These kinds of insults happen to regular people all the time and probably much more often than you are likely to be aware, absenting your conscious attention for them.

Quite often these insults, when they happen on an isolated and non-recurring basis, will not contribute in any significant way to your eventual decline. For example, a poor night's sleep can usually be made up for the next night; a hangover following the annual New Year's Eve party will probably not shave years from your life; if ever you incur a stiff neck you may be able to work out the kinks without lasting ill effect. But if poor sleep or over-indulgence is the rule rather than the exception, or if your stiff neck persists or recurs on a regular basis, that redefines both the nature, and the effect, of the insult. I repeat: it is the cumulative effect of a multitude of minor insults over time that causes them to become problematic.

Norman Doidge, M.D., described how neural real estate is allotted on a priority basis according to the demand for its use. "...when we learn a bad habit, it takes over a brain map, and each time we repeat it, it claims more control of that map and prevents the use of that space for 'good' habits. That is why 'unlearning' is often harder than learning...."[7] Though Doidge was specifically referring to the acquisition of language skills, he was also describing perfectly the process by which insults against the body culminate as new and errant default settings in the brain, and why, once embedded, the effects of insults can be so challenging to dismantle.

Next, after minor level insults, we move up a notch to "medium level" insults. Medium level insults are rarer than minor insults, yet not at all uncommon. A sampling of this level of insult might include sprains and strains such as a turned ankle or a back spasm, jarring and bruises from sporting or recreational activities, a slip on the ice that bruises your coccyx, a slow-to-resolve emotional trauma, or repeated challenges on the limits of the body's abilities. We all incur medium level insults; but, by comparison, these occur less frequently, perhaps only a few times a year, if you're lucky, rather than many times daily as with lesser insults. Unlike minor issues such as those on the first level, the effects of medium level insults can linger, either overtly as in the case of a sprained ankle that heals slowly, or less obviously as simmering emotional concerns, or perhaps as a back spasm that subsides but remains susceptible to flaring up again when triggered by stressors.

Notably, minor insults can transform into medium level problems, as when a benign act like toting a handbag or a child shifts from an occasional experience to part of a regular or daily pattern, or when that stiff neck doesn't go away. Dean Juhan described this propensity in *Job's Body* when he asserted, "...locomotor patterns become individualized by one's unique pattern of experiences..." Regarding the body, he noted, "...repeated gestures become postures, and sustained postures become structures." Regarding the mind, he added, "An oft repeated mental event becomes a tendency, a tendency followed long enough becomes a habit, and a habit exercised long enough becomes a bit of personal identity."[8] The idea that people can become habitu-

---

7   Norman Doidge M.D., *The Brain That Changes Itself*. Viking, 2007.
8   Dean Juhan, *Job's Body*. Barrytown/Station Hill, 2003.

ated to their actions (and inured to the effects of those actions) was elucidated by William James in 1890 when he wrote, "A tendency to act only becomes effectively ingrained in us in proportion to the uninterrupted frequency with which the actions actually occur, and the brain 'grows' to their use."[9] Thus can issues of minor concern escalate to a level of greater concern.

An unlikely example of how a seemingly innocuous behavior can shift into a medium level insult presented itself in one of my Taijiquan students. This gentleman had the habit of scrunching his neck somewhat forward rather than holding his head properly erect (clearly a medium level insult), and as a result had been struggling for some time to integrate my advice during Tai Chi practice that he position his head and neck in a more anatomically correct manner. It dawned on him one day, just as our class was finishing up a round of somatics movement patterns, that his bifocal glasses were implicated in his postural discrepancy. Apparently, his glasses caused him to adopt the habit of scrunching his neck whenever he sought to focus his vision, which, of course, he did repeatedly throughout the day. His glasses not only created a minor insult initially, but over time they served to reinforce and exacerbate the errant pattern that resulted, and even to stymie his best attempts at correcting it.

Finally, we have a level of "major insults." This more severe level would be comprised of badly broken bones, major surgeries, automobile accidents, stress caused by failed marriages or ruined careers, strokes, etc. These can be hurts that not only last, but which serve to redefine our sense of personal identity. Insults such as these may only occur once every five or ten years or so (again, a generalized assumption offered just for the sake of illustration). Despite their infrequent occurrence for most people, the effects of major insults can be devastating.

---

9 William James, *The Principles of Psychology,* Vol. 1. Cosimo Classics, 1890.

It All Adds Up

Different individuals will be more or less susceptible or fortunate in the nature and frequency of the insults they incur. Someone with a more sedentary lifestyle, perhaps a writer, may be more inclined toward low level insults, while a construction worker or sports enthusiast may be more prone toward medium level bumps and bruises. Riskier lifestyles, obviously, entail more risk, but medium to severe level insults are often unpredictable in form and fashion and can hit anyone any time. Just as obviously, people will vary in their response to, and resilience against, various insults and stressors. That said, let's consider some purely hypothetical statistics so that you might reflect on the numbers of minor, medium level, and major insults that someone experiences *in toto* over the course of a typical lifetime.

Minor insults probably occur dozens of times each day for most people. For the sake of argument allow me to (very conservatively) estimate three insults per day. Over the course of a year, that adds up to a thousand insults. Add in a couple of medium level insults each year; and over the course of a decade you've got ten thousand minor insults, plus several dozen medium level insults, and maybe some really major event as well. Remember, this is your body we're talking about. Multiply these figures by five, or six, or seven decades, if you happen to be middle-aged or older, and you start to get the picture: the cumulative picture of a person whose body is well advanced beyond the freedom and ease of youth, and stumbling headlong toward the discomfort, inflexibility, and systemic decline so characteristic of old age.

I reiterate that not every insult has lasting or equal consequences, and that the body has remarkable regenerative powers in its ability to self-repair in many cases. Nevertheless, I feel that I've been extremely conservative in understating the figures cited above. Even if we were to arbitrarily reduce these figures further, say by fifty percent, we're still talking about tens of thousands of insults against your body over the course of a few decades. That's a lot of insults! The average body responds to the onslaught painted above with adaptation and resilience where it can, but eventually the weight of this archeology comes to bear on your body in the form of pathological reflex patterns evidencing senile degeneration and decline.

As if all this weren't cause enough for concern, physiologic decline carries with it the likelihood of reduced self-efficacy. The damage wrought by the embodied myth of aging is insidious in its effects on our non-physiologic selves as well. As the body comes gradually to experience less and less freedom in the manner in which it organizes and expresses itself, our belief system about ourselves becomes correspondingly limited. That is, our self-image, in its own best attempt to maintain some sense of personal congruity, readjusts to reflect (and thereby reinforce) the experience we have of our bodies. Bodies that become less able to move freely invite the mindsets they house to become correspondingly constrained, thus becoming invested in that loss of ability. "I'm not as young as I used to be," "I guess I'm just getting older," and, "You can't teach an old dog new tricks," are all-too-common statements of belief that reflect and reinforce the myth of aging. We observe our diminishing freedom and so come to think that we *can't* be as free, and that this *must* be what it's like to grow old; and we fulfill the prophesy.

You might reasonably ask, "How can this happen in our age of modern technology?" or "Why doesn't science or medicine point their spotlight on this to fix it?" or, on a more personal level, "How can this happen to me?" After all, science has us getting upwards of forty miles per gallon on many cars; technology has us getting stock quotes and movies on our cell phones, and we've been to the moon. In light of these and other advances, the issue of addressing debilitating insults to alleviate the full sweep of human pain and suffering believed to be caused by aging ought to be both a breeze and something of a priority, at least on the order of moon-walking, gas mileage, and personal finance.

The answer is complicated because aging is now big business that is getting bigger. The simplest explanation is that nearly everybody buys into "the myth." We've all been indoctrinated to expect that aging culminates in a predictable decline. Plus, our culture is heavily invested, both economically and belief system-wise, in services (Medicare, Medicaid) and products (pharmaceuticals, retirement facilities, etc.) that target pain and chronic disease— arthritis, back pain, headaches, digestive disturbances, respiratory ailments, hypertension, cardiovascular issues, allergies, erectile dysfunction, etc.

One need only glance at the various visual media (Internet, magazines, newspapers, TV) or at the amount of shelf space devoted to analgesics in your local pharmacy, to get a sense of how pervasive this mindset is. Scientific and medical entities that are profit-based, not to mention insurance entities, have a big stake in this status quo. Imagine if it could be shown that even a moderate percentage of erectile dysfunction sufferers could find some measure of relief in a few simple movement patterns. Can you imagine Pfizer and Lilly pulling Viagra and Cialis (replete with their "afterthought warnings" about priapism) from the shelves and, instead, spending millions of dollars to research simple exercise patterns that cannot be patented, packaged, or sold? Or, in the same vein, what if it could be shown that headaches or backaches could be avoided or managed in a similarly simple fashion, obviating the need for the smorgasbord of pain medications whose marketing campaigns compete incessantly for our attention?[10]

Conventional medicine, which prides itself on being scientific, has been anything but scientific in identifying and addressing the underlying causes of age-related neuromuscular degeneration. Medical professionals and scientists alike have long been as presumptuous about the degenerative effects of aging on the body as has the general populace. In all fairness to conventional medicine, the ultimate responsibility for avoiding or correcting problems stemming from the archeology of insults lies not with the government or with any other agency, but with each and every individual person. Herein we have a large part of the appeal of somatic education. In addition to its efficacy, HSE can be learned or

---

10 Lest you dismiss my cynicism toward institutional entities as singular and unwarranted, you might consider that author Michael Pollan draws a strikingly similar inference in his 2008 book, *In Defense of Food*, p. 141.

experienced quickly and easily, not to mention relatively cheaply, by anybody.

Thomas Hanna offered up a solution which is so simple and widely accessible that one would expect the claims made by Hanna and those who ascribe to his approach to arouse the passions of skeptics and quack-busters everywhere. The plain fact of the matter is that somatic education has its basis in simple, yet indisputable, science. The theories on which somatics is based are founded in conventional neurophysiology; and its claims, albeit empirical at this writing, are supported by clinical experience. Despite the hint of mystique suggested by such catch phrases as the "myth of aging" and the "archeology of insults" there is nothing about somatics that is even remotely faith-based or New-Agey, however low-tech it may be. Continuing advances in the neurosciences only serve to reinforce the most basic premises of somatics.

The passage of time is unavoidable; and insults such as we have discussed are, for all practical purposes, part of the human condition. Yet somatics provides us some measure of recourse. The goal of somatics is to help people learn how to exercise and assert the cortical brain's conscious control over the body's neuromuscular system, and to disarm and dismantle the effects of the archeology of insults responsible for declines in neuromuscular efficiency (including pain, stiffness, postural imbalances, etc.).

Somatic education accomplishes this task by recruiting the conscious and voluntary attention of the cortical brain to recalibrate the errant default settings of the sub-cortical brain. Such recalibration serves to restore optimal communication via the sensorimotor pathways with chronically engaged muscles, so that they may finally stand down and relax. Thus is fuller and more efficient voluntary control over the body's neuromuscular system restored, and with it a renewed quality of life.

CHAPTER 2

WHAT ARE THE BENEFITS OF SOMATICS?

Longer Muscles

Among the claims made by proponents of somatic education is that somatics can help achieve improved flexibility. Almost everyone, even persons not of a "fitness persuasion," equates flexibility with freedom—freedom of one's body—and rightfully so; because decreased flexibility augurs debility and decline. In my own practices, I have certainly found merit to this claim. Having more than forty years experience as a martial arts teacher, I have witnessed such improvement firsthand in my Tai Chi and Kung Fu classes where I frequently integrate somatic movement patterns into the warm-up or cool-down phase of classes. I see comparable improvements in my clinical setting, working with ordinary people who fall well outside the martial arts stereotype. In either case, immediate changes in flexibility, though on occasion quite obvious and dramatic, vary according to factors specific to the client, and also according to the protocol[1] or movement patterns chosen for the occasion.

However, even though improved flexibility does result from experiencing somatics, flexibility, as such, is not our primary goal in working with clients, not if it is achieved in lieu of more intelligence in the muscles. More on this shortly.

There are many ways to make muscles longer, as evidenced by the vast numbers of approaches catering to this goal. Many of these methods rely on aggressive or forcible lengthening of muscles. Approaches that entail forced stretching usually produce results that are both superficial and temporary.

---

1   HSE protocols entail a prearranged sequence of teaching methods and maneuvers designed to address patterns of habituation, e.g., Red Light, Green Light, or Trauma reflex, according to Thomas Hanna's design. See Chapter 3.

Forcible stretching can also prove counterproductive in directly causing or precipitating injury, or in eliciting the body's stretch reflex.[2] Younger bodies may seem more amenable to aggressive stretching—and to a certain degree they are—but mostly that's because younger bodies have not, typically, yet become as saddled with the effects of sensorimotor amnesia.

In any attempt to lengthen muscles that have become unnaturally tight or chronically contracted, the most sensible method of all is to first simply eliminate whatever causative factors are responsible for muscles being contracted in the first place. To paraphrase Thomas Hanna, the purpose of somatics is to teach people how to regain sensory awareness of those muscles that have become unconsciously and involuntarily contracted, *in order to regain that degree of voluntary control (and flexibility) that has been lost.*[3] This, then, is our primary goal as somatics educators—to recoup that which has been lost, before concerning ourselves with any net gain. It makes little sense to force-stretch a tight muscle if only to activate the stretch reflex that re-contracts that same muscle. Trying to coerce a contracted muscle into a relaxed, i.e. longer, state is tantamount to fomenting internal conflict within your own body. Why engage in conflict if there's an easier way?

Somatics offers the prospect of an easier way. Instead of entering into conflict by trying to force a contracted muscle longer, the somatics approach is to work with muscles rather than against them. By adopting this approach, we enhance the likelihood of developing muscles that are "smarter" as well as longer. When muscles are smart (meaning their communication with the brain via the sensorimotor pathways has not been compromised), baseline flexibility will naturally ensue. Whatever additional flexibility one might gain as a result of a somatics experience is simply icing on the cake of more intelligent muscles.

---

2 The Stretch Reflex, aka myotatic reflex, is the body's simplest (monosynaptic reflex arc) reflex response, i.e., contracts an over-stretched muscle or tendon.
3 Thomas Hanna's archived lectures, CD # 34, July 17, 1990.

Despite the uniform design of our human anatomy,[4] no two bodies are exactly the same in terms of physiologic potential. I recall some thirty or so years ago working out at my Kung Fu school with a then-local colleague, Billy Blanks (of Tae Bo fame). Billy was a fighter *extraordinaire*, and at the time I happened to be the reigning regional forms champion. Billy and I got together every now and then for practice at my school, each of us sharing tips to help the other. I recall on one occasion, as we were warming up before practice, watching in awe as Billy just dropped into a full split. Ouch! Meanwhile, I just happened to be casually reaching with my elbow down along the front of my unbent front leg to touch elbow-to-toe. I wasn't really paying attention to myself as I was so taken with Billy's flexibility. I was surprised, therefore, when he glanced over at me and said, "Man, how do you do that?" This has ever served as a reminder to me of how different bodies each have their own potentialities.

Smarter Muscles

Naturally, the goals of somatics, in its most global sense, are to ease human pain and suffering and to help you realize your greatest potential for freedom in your own body. Gaining "smarter" muscles is the means by which we accomplish both of these goals. While there is no brain or brain equivalent in the muscles,[5] any upper-echelon athlete (think here of the likes of Roger Federer, Michael Jordan, Serena Williams, or Rudolf Nureyev—for whom "body intelligence" is preeminent) instinctively knows that his or her body and brain must work together in perfect harmony for peak performance. Peak performance requires a certain quality of neuromuscular intelligence.

"Intelligence" is defined as the "capacity for learning, reasoning and

---

4   Congenital defect and occasional anomalies aside, all humans have the same muscles and bones.
5   In seeming contradiction of this, The History Channel's program, *The Brain*, 11/10/08, reported new evidence suggesting there may be an actual mechanism for memory in the muscles.

understanding... aptitude for grasping facts, meanings, etc."[6] Usually such qualities are ascribed solely to the brain, which conventional and prevailing wisdom credits for intelligence and memory storage. While the brain may represent our "hard drive," responsible for facilitating all our different "software applications," our brain is only as useful and practical as the computer "hardware" (the body) in which it is installed. For practical purposes, it is the congruity between the brain and body, not just in terms of communication efficiency but also in terms of performance potential, that determines how well and how extensively the body is able to function in the environment. No matter how smart the brain is, it still needs cooperation and compliance from muscles if it is to get anything done. Exactly what quality and degree of cooperation and compliance the brain gets from our muscles depends on their ability to perform.

This is where "differentiation" enters the picture, because intelligence in our muscles is measured in how well they can respond (perform) to our brains' dictates. Muscles that have had more, or less, experience will have a corresponding degree of representation in the brain. As early as the 1920s, Karl Lashley determined that muscles receive cortical representation according to the demands for their use.[7] Well-differentiated muscles warrant more cortical real estate. Though our muscles may not be smart in any cognitive sense, there is certainly plenty of room for performance variation in how effectively they function as vehicles for the brain's intelligence. If our brain asks for precise or methodical movement and the muscles fail to respond exactly as directed, well, let's just say they won't qualify as Mensa muscles. If, on the other hand, our muscles do exactly what the brain directs them to do, we've got Ivy League muscles.

In (simple) neurological terms, what this entails is optimal functioning of the body's sensorimotor system. Afferent pathways provide information to the

---

6 *Random House Webster's College Dictionary.* 1992.
7 Jeffery M. Schwartz M.D. and Sharon Begley, *The Mind and The Brain.* ReganBooks, 2002.

brain; and efferent tracks, in turn, carry "do this" impulses from the brain to the motor system. If something transpires to impede the flow of information to the brain, i.e., a muscle becomes chronically contracted in a learned reflex pattern due to injury or overuse, the brain is deprived of a critical component in its ability to communicate effectively with the body. The brain becomes, in effect, amnesiac to that muscle, or whatever portion of the muscle is remiss in its motor function. Lacking sensory input from the forgotten muscle, the brain has no basis, or reason, for correcting a problem it doesn't know exists. To put it in the vernacular, the muscle becomes stupid.

This "stupidity" has two components, rendering it a two-phase problem. First, as the brain is deprived of critical feedback, it adjusts its default setting for muscle tonus accordingly; so that as far as the brain is concerned the effects of debilitating sensorimotor amnesia (expressed as chronic hypertonus) in that muscle become the norm. Second, because of the ensuing disuse of the motor tracks involved, dendrites[8] stemming from the neurons that serve compromised muscle are decommissioned. This pruning process[9] results in a decline in dendritic density and a corresponding reduction in synaptic junctures, known in neuro-speak as "long-term synaptic depression." The natural tendency of the brain to all this (the shadow side, if you will, of neuroplasticity), is not to repair the problem *in situ*, but to reallocate its resources elsewhere rather than maintain dendrites and synapses that are inactive. It's always a seller's market in the brain, so reallocation of resources all too often takes precedence over fixing what's "broken." According to Sharon Begley, "Cortical real estate that used to serve one purpose is reassigned and begins to do another. The brain remakes itself, in response to outside stimuli—to its environment and to experience."[10] The decline in dendritic density and synaptic allocation thus reinforces the sensorimotor amnesia, and so on, in a

---

8 Dendrites are the nerve receptors on neurons that collect or receive information for passage along from neuron to neuron.
9   This is not to be confused with *apoptosis*, which is a programmed and developmentally appropriate pruning of neurons that occurs at predetermined growth stages.
10 Sharon Begley, *Train Your Mind to Change Your Brain*. Ballantine, 2007.

continuing cycle that culminates in a *fait accompli* of pain or restricted movement, à la your typical senile posture.

However, the very act of trying to use a muscle in a conscious and deliberate manner can have just the opposite effect. Your regular and repeated attempts at deliberate and methodical movement increase the concentration of dendrites and synapses according to the new or renewed demand for the service they provide. This proliferation of dendrites provides the basis for restoring old learning tracks or creating new ones, in effect interrupting the "stupid" cycle and resetting the brain's default mechanism for motor function. The new or renewed sensorimotor learning tracks, in facilitating enhanced neuromuscular communication, now provide the basis for smarter muscles as evidenced by more differentiated movement. From here on, we just have to keep our muscles smart.

Sustainability

One of the great catch phrases of our time is sustainability. We hear talk of sustainability in regards to energy and environmental issues, from fossil fuel depletion and renewable resources such as wind or solar power to the lumber industry and organic farming. We also find that term applied in other contexts, such as troop preparedness and infrastructure for military scenarios, as well as in regard to political ideologies or agendas. In a similar vein, we have another popular adjective currently in vogue—green—which rightly or wrongly has been employed as an association word, much like the words "organic" or "natural" to imply that something is somehow healthier or lower impact in its negative or nonrenewable effects on the earth and those who populate it.

I maintain that there are no contexts in which the concept of sustainability, or of being green, is more personally relevant than with regard to our own health. In Chapter 1 we discussed how different levels of insults could be attributed to a wide range of causes, any of which boded the prospect of some degree of "net loss" to our health and wellness. Even those activities or experiences not considered to be outright bad for us may merely prove break-even, or neutral, i.e. a tradeoff, in their aftereffects.

Somatic education, on the other hand, is one of a very limited number of wellness resources that offers any compelling prospect of "net gain," meaning that we receive substantially more of a return on our investment of time and energy than the expenditure we put out in achieving that gain. How green is that! In short, somatics is good for you for personal sustainability.

Most people spend the greater part of their lives working at a trade, or building a career, or attending to family, etc. In doing so it's easy to lose sight of the fact that we work to live, and not vice versa. Altogether too many people "live to work," or are devoted excessively to some extrinsic cause at great personal cost. Those who slip into this trap—and in doing so forget how to meet their own needs in a fundamentally sustainable way—court the myth of aging and all its decline. Somatic education is a means of personal sustenance and renewal—of living green, so to speak—that enables us to assume control of our own life from within and altogether separately from external circumstances.

With Freedom Comes Responsibility

Any shift toward sustainability requires that we comport ourselves in a sustainable manner. Therefore, a standard part of the somatics experience entails a personal maintenance program. Regardless of whether we have simply learned a series of somatics movement patterns, or have worked in a hands-on setting with a trained somatic educator, we must assume responsibility for continually reinforcing what the body has learned. The effects of hands-on table work[11] can be immediate and dramatic in many cases, depending on variables specific to your body and its condition. Alternatively, movement pattern practices can also produce sometimes rapid results. Typically, though, the effects derived solely from movement pattern practices may not be as expedient or as dramatic as when you work with a somatic educator directly. In either case, whether practicing movement patterns alone or in follow-up to a clinical session, the beneficial effects experienced will accrue on a cumulative basis as the brain and body collaborate toward a more differentiated movement.

As with most other endeavors, the more you practice at something the more skilled you become at it. Regular practice enables you to more aptly discern the finer points of whatever you practice. This is certainly the case with somatics as you gradually improve your ability over time to sense and control your own body at finer and finer increments of differentiation. However, the responsibility to comply with whatever follow-up advice is given by your chosen provider remains yours, as no one other than yourself can connect the dots between your brain and your motor system. Freedom and sustainability don't just happen on their own; they must be achieved and actively maintained.

Methodical and Differentiated, Versus Momentum-based Movement

To be truly in command of your body and how it moves you must be capable of methodical movement,[12] movement that is slow, meticulous, and mindful. Practicing at methodical movement will improve your ability to move your body in a precisely differentiated manner. Differentiation, here, implies the ability to sense and control the movements of your body deliberately and purposefully in the absence of impediments preventing you from doing so. In somatics we encourage clients to move slowly and methodically so that they'll

---

11 Some somatic educators prefer to position their clients on a mat on the floor rather than on a table for individual sessions.

12 Methodical movement facilitates an enhanced sense of *what* moves and *how,* known in somatics as the *means whereby.*

not be deprived, due to any inadvertent reliance on momentum, of any opportunity for self-sensing.

Regardless of the specific terminology, movement that is methodical requires a combination of attention and intention and an absence of inadvertent momentum. Momentum that is inadvertent is the very antithesis of differentiated movement. Imagine a stereotypical elderly person in a debilitated state, someone whose balance has declined to a point that they are stumbling, shuffling, or lurching about; you have in that person an extreme example of movement that is undifferentiated, methodically imprecise, and inappropriately reliant on, or subject to, momentum. Such momentum, especially in the presence of an inability to move in a balanced and controlled manner from one's center, is the primary reason why older folks are so notoriously susceptible to falls. Sadly, undifferentiated movement is far more common than with just the occasional elderly person, or even the elderly population in general, where the absence of differentiation is so clearly evident in its culminating phase.

The more sobering reality is that most people begin to lose their ability to move with methodical precision and clear-cut differentiation at a much earlier age. The postures that typify blatant senile debilitation are, in most cases, nothing more than the cumulative results of a life lived, and often have roots in behaviors or experiences tracing all the way back to one's youth. As a lifelong martial arts teacher, I've had the opportunity to closely observe the developing bodies of quite a few of my young charges as they matured, many from preschool age through to fully developed adult bodies. I know from my own direct observations that errant patterns in adults often announce themselves at least as early as four or five years of age.[13]

To repeat: movement based on inadvertent momentum is mindless movement. In fact, momentum-based movement is a compensation for being

---

13 This brings to mind the rather radical conjecture that postural dissonance can stem at an early age from social osmosis, as children may adopt postures modeled after influential others who, themselves, suffer the effects of sensorimotor amnesia.

mind-*less* about your movement. Anytime you don't think about your movement it becomes just that—mindless. Practically speaking, you can't always be consciously aware of what your body is doing at all times. You'd never get anything else accomplished. From your brain's perspective, at any given moment millions of sensory stimuli are all clamoring for its attention. Fortunately, filtering mechanisms prioritize stimuli so that we're not constantly overwhelmed by sensory minutia. However, barring any impediments, e.g., faulty filtering mechanisms, it is in developing your ability to be *electively* mindful that your full potential for methodical and differentiated movement can be applied.

Add In Proprioception and Implicit Memory

Because the brain is bombarded by an unceasing flow of sensory data, much of it irrelevant to our immediate safety and well-being, evolution has developed mechanisms by which we remain functional even without a hundred percent conscious attention. For younger people "in their prime," so to speak, the body and the brain's ability to function relatively mindlessly, or automatically, is made possible in part by an innate and seamless collaboration between implicit memory and proprioceptive function. Implicit memory is generally unconscious and, though not limited to motor function, certainly plays a major role in many of the activities we perform with our bodies without thinking, such as walking or running, or other repetitive and automatic tasks and behaviors.

Proprioception is the process by which a continuous flow of sensory feedback messages from nerve sensors strategically located throughout the body reach the brain, informing it about the body's spatial organization. Between the neural transactions of implicit memory and proprioceptive feedback there is quite a lot going on in the brain.[14] "Quite a lot" makes for a bit of an under-

---

14 This simplistic model does not even factor in data from the vestibular nuclei, which offer their own contribution to balance.

statement as these events happen according to a potentially incalculable speed and magnitude.[15] The brain in turn, and based on this input of information, tells the body what to do, how to respond or behave or adjust. This is why, if we are younger and relatively healthy, we need not think about putting one foot forward of the other while walking, even on uneven terrain, or while performing any of a thousand other daily tasks on automatic pilot.

> However, there's a catch to this process. The catch is that this automatic pilot system only works reliably as long as there is a continuous flow of revealing and accurate information passed along to the brain. If anything should occur to impede the flow of accurate information to the brain its ability to seamlessly control and direct the body becomes compromised.

Unfortunately, impediments to the flow of sensory information to the brain are common, even pandemic. Such impediments, caused by the same insults discussed in the previous chapter, are the true cause of what most people experience as age-related declines in balance, flexibility, and overall freedom of movement. This is precisely what is implied by "the myth of aging." This catch phrase, coined by Thomas Hanna and now a part of the somatics lexicon, encapsulates his views on the typical aging process.

Thus, it is not really aging *per se* that causes the greater range of debilitating neuromuscular symptoms commonly associated with getting older. Aging, itself, simply sets the stage for sensorimotor amnesia as the longer we're alive the more time and opportunity we have to experience insults that cause debilitation. The real cause of neuromuscular debilitation is a progressive de-

---

15 Bernard J. Baars, *In the Theater of Consciousness*, Oxford Univ. Press, 1997. The brain is able to process up to 6,000,000,000,000 (6 trillion) events per second. Jeffery Schwartz M.D. and Sharon Begley go one better in their 2002 book, *The Mind and the Brain*, alleging somewhere on the order of 100–1,000 trillion synapses in the adult brain! Of course, they don't all fire at once, and not every synaptic event involves proprioception, motor function, or implicit memory. But the "incalculable speed and magnitude" qualification above seems conservative enough, given the numbers.

cline in the brain's ability to compensate for inefficient and insufficient sensory input. Poor sensory input undermines the brain's basis for appropriate motor output. Faulty wiring, so to speak, with our implicit, aka procedural, memories can compound this situation.

Put another way: If you had a late model car with all the latest computer sensors designed to pinpoint system failures, but the computer sensors themselves failed to work properly, would you blame your car's ensuing mechanical problems on the car for being too old? Of course not, because the underlying cause of the problems is not the car's age. Knowing this, would you then tow your vehicle off to the junkyard? Not likely. You would take steps to repair the faulty sensors. Once the sensors were restored to working order you would have every reason to expect the car to perform according to its engineered potential. This is exactly the approach we take in somatics, recalibrating the body's computer hard drive sensors through methodical movement. Methodical movement, applied during certain patterns and positions mapped out by somatics educators, is designed to restore your computer sensors to full working order so you can drive like a Mercedes, instead of a beat-up old pick-up truck. Methodical movement is the means by which you develop the ability to differentiate and control the muscles of your body, perhaps to a level of nuance.

But, you might ask, what if you are younger and regard yourself as relatively healthy and in control of your body? Can *you* benefit from somatics? Even if you are younger and well able to operate on automatic pilot, just because you can do so doesn't necessarily mean you should *only* do so. Somatics is not just for older people. It is never too early in life to get into the good habit of methodical movement to optimize your proprioceptive function. Like changing your car's oil, a little bit of preventative maintenance can go a long way in helping you to avert future problems. Even a Mercedes requires preventative maintenance.

Think of methodical movement as akin to meditation. Meditation is what conduces us or lulls us into the moment at hand, to be more fully present to ourselves and more aware of our own ongoing internal processes.

Meditation is popularly regarded as a mental (or spiritual) experience, albeit one that can affect the physical self. It is old news that meditation can have a measurable, even dramatic, effect on the physical body. However, this is often seen as a one-way street as scant consideration is given to the corollary, that the body can substantively affect the mind beyond simply reducing the perceived effects of stress or depression. In many circles it would sound curious indeed to hear of someone "meditating their body" to calm their mind.

John Ratey M.D. echoed this sentiment in *Spark* when he stated, "...the idea that we can alter our mental state by physically moving still has yet to be accepted by most physicians, let alone the broader public."[16] Yet it's no stretch to say that the experience of feeling as if one's body has been "meditated" is one of the more delightful effects of engaging in the practice of somatics. Nowhere is it etched in stone that the beneficial effects of meditation on the body can't work in reverse. A meditated body is perfectly capable of conducing its effects on the brain. In fact, the effects on your mind of carefully orchestrated body movements that are truly methodical can be indistinguishable from the effects of meditation. What happens to our body happens to our brain, and vice versa.

Listening to Your Body

In Taijiquan, an art and discipline that I have practiced and taught since the mid-1970s, there are both solo practice features and interactive aspects. For cooperative practices in which two individuals engage in prearranged or spontaneous practice routines involving contact (touch), a quality known as ting jin is highly regarded. Ting jin literally translates as "listening skill"; but instead of listening with one's ears, ting jin implies listening via one's sense of touch, feeling for an opponent's intention or weakness in a manner seemingly intuitive. The implications of ting jin are somewhat analogous to the

---

16   Ratey adds, "The advantage of using exercise to inoculate the brain against stress is that it ramps up growth factors more than other stimuli do. In addition to being produced in the brain...(growth factors) are also generated by muscle contractions and then travel...into the brain to further support neurons."

Western concept of "reading between the lines," to perceive that which is not readily perceivable, only applied in Tai Chi as bodily sensitivity as opposed to intuition or deductive reasoning.

In Tai Chi, ting jin skill may require years of diligent practice to fully develop. Once developed, its acquisition indicates the achievement of an advanced level of skill at Taijiquan. The acquisition of ting jin starts with setting a stage conducive to listening and then simply practicing at same, paying attention for that which is difficult to perceive. To quote Dr. Jay Dunbar, a Tai Chi colleague, "Expertise consists in being able to differentiate between subtly different situations or conditions."[17] This is just another way of saying that self-mastery stems from practicing at differentiation. It follows that the key to acquiring Tai Chi's ting jin skill starts with creating the right conditions for its development.

Regarding the human body, only the rare person knows how to self-sense, to really listen deeply within. Some people are able to develop some aspects of their self-sensing potential through meditation. But when they listen, what are they likely to hear? Methodical movement such as we ascribe to in somatics goes beyond mental awareness. It tunes us in, primarily, to our state of body, as well as our mind. We would do well to remember that self-sensing is about more than just motor behavior. It is also about interfacing our very capacity for motor behavior with our inner subjective perception of self. A hallmark of somatics is that we encourage clients to hone their ability for noticing, interoceptively, to increase their level of somato-sensory awareness.

An inherent feature common to both somatics and Tai Chi is that each discipline is so elegant in its simplicity that both entail doing less in order to accomplish more. The great irony lies in how challenging it can be to keep it simple. With Tai Chi and somatics, the hardest part is in making it easy.

---

17 John Loupos, *Exploring Tai Chi—Contemporary Views on an Ancient Art*, YMAA Publications. 2002.

Just as in Tai Chi, the way we begin to accomplish this with somatics is by creating an environment conducive to such awareness. Not an external environment, but our internal one. As with Taijiquan, this is best accomplished by moving slowly, so as not to fall into any mode of automatic pilot in which momentum displaces conscious awareness of one's actions and behavior. Slow movement creates an ideal opportunity for self-sensing because methodical slowness requires a departure from the mesmerizing cadence of inadvertent momentum that governs and defines most people's lives.

Author Louis Cozolino notes, in the context of psychotherapy, that powerful shifts in self-awareness are often characterized by clients verbalizing their thoughts more slowly due to the added challenge of organizing sentences when not relying on semantic habits and clichés, in other words, when they are deprived of verbal momentum.[18] Slowing down allows us to become aware of and observe aspects of the self—of the mind and body both—that would otherwise escape conscious scrutiny.

To draw on another automotive analogy, I liken this to driving your car along the highway. At sixty mph you may think you are taking in all the scenery that the roadside has to offer. However, if you park the car and meander along the same roadside you'll surely notice many details you simply could not have perceived at the faster pace, even though those same details were there all along. Noticing the internal details of your own body as you meander daily along your own roadside is one of the keys to sustainable health and well-being.

Along these lines, it bears mentioning that any preexisting experiences one has at somatics or other methods of self-sensing have limited value as inactive assets. Whatever somatics movement patterns or clinical work you may have previously engaged in to address past problems will have little bearing on future problems that may crop up. Future problems that may occur will call for their own somatics work. I've had previously discharged clients

---

18 Louis Cozolino, *The Neuroscience of Psychotherapy.* Norton, 2002.

return to report that this or that problem cropped back up under duress, only to reveal under questioning that, "no," they haven't been keeping up their home practice exercises. It's not enough that you did somatics, you must do somatics on a regular basis.

Taking the position that last week's exercises are sufficient to avoid tomorrow's problems is an ill advised strategy. You must meander along your roadside each and every day to stay abreast of the changing details of your own life.

More on Proprioceptive Literacy

Proprioceptive literacy implies the brain's ability to sense and know where its body is in relationship to itself and to its environment at any given time, and to enact whatever changes or adjustments may be called for to ensure that the body and brain maintain an optimally collaborative relationship. Proprioception, ideally, entails both having that information and being able to act on it.[19]

All the aforementioned benefits and techniques—longer muscles, smarter muscles, methodical movements, and self-sensing—contribute to, and stem from, an increase in proprioceptive literacy. These are mutually reinforcing dynamics. For many people, enhanced proprioceptive literacy is the very "pot-o-gold" waiting for those who ascribe to the somatics approach to neuromuscular wellness. Proprioceptive literacy is what we inadvertently surrender as the effects of sensorimotor amnesia ravage our bodies over time, decade after decade. And proprioceptive literacy is exactly what you stand to (re)gain as your brain learns how to reassert control over the muscles in its domain.

Many of the latest neurophysiological findings support this line of thought. New developments in the neurosciences continue to reveal intricacies about brain function and performance in shedding light on what is

19 Usually proprioception is regarded as a sensory function. My use of the term "proprioceptive literacy" implies the brain's ability to match sensory feedback with a desired motor program.

understood to be possible for the human brain and, by extension, for the body it oversees. For example, a team of researchers at the Netherlands Institute for Brain Research determined that ongoing and regular activation of selected brain areas may prevent or delay degenerative effects in those particular areas of the brain.[20] This hypothesis was supported in findings by British scientists showing that a part of the brain believed to be involved in spatial learning and memory, known as the hippocampus, was demonstrably larger in a sampling of sixteen London cab drivers as compared to a fifty member control group and, furthermore, to be proportionately larger according to the number of years a cabbie had been on the job.[21]

In another experiment done at the University of California at Irvine, researchers working with rats showed that exercise actually encourages growth of hippocampal memory cells.[22] Assuming these findings apply to humans as well, we might surmise that exercise, and particularly mindful exercise, ala somatics, helps to shape a part of the neural architecture that has bearing on motor sequence memory. If it is true that activation of selected brain areas contributes to the growth and performance of cognitive abilities, then perhaps it is not too great a leap to hypothesize that regular and focused use of those parts of the brain that control proprioception and motor function might be similarly amenable to preservation and even improvement, or at least retarded decline. This has yet to be proven, but much of what we now know and accept as being true and scientifically valid in many aspects of science and medicine merely confirms what we've long experienced as empirically valid. Sometimes science just has to play catch-up with common sense.

Somatic education is not a panacea. Nor does it present itself as a fountain of youth in which the clock is foiled. Yet, somatics can offer the best of several worlds—as a cognitive activity that fortifies both brain function and

---

20 Elkhonon Goldberg, *The Executive Brain*. Oxford, 2001. Citation of Mirmiran, van Someren, and Swaab, *Behav. Brain Res* 78, # 1 (96).

21 Maguire, et al. "Navigation-related structural change in the hippocampi of taxi drivers," *Proc Natl Acad Sci USA* 97, #8 (2000).

22 Jeff Victoroff, M.D., *Saving Your Brain*. Bantom Books, 2002.

body fitness, and as a physical exercise that simultaneously reinforces body fitness and brain function. Somatics contradicts the long-held dictum that "structure (alone) creates function." We now know that the corollary—that "function begets structure"—is every bit as true. This means that each of us, to quote Thomas Hanna, "...is largely responsible for who and what we become." Somatics offers you the possibility of avoiding unnecessary or premature decline and debilitation of body and brain, and the means by which you can accomplish a quality of personal maintenance for yourself, and by yourself, without expensive, intrusive, or risky third party interventions.

Imagine a future in which your body feels or behaves as if it were years younger than the bodies of your peers, affording both freedom from pain and the added freedom of mobility. What you are imagining can be a reality whose time for you has come. You need only get yourself started to enjoy these benefits and more.

CHAPTER 3

SOMATIC PROTOCOLS

Three Perspectives

A basic presumption in somatics is that the center or core of the body (meaning the trunk or torso, and including the waist), necessarily affects the entire rest of the body. Thus, the initial assumption of a trained somatic educator is that any attempt to redress neuromuscular imbalances must start from the core. Even though a client might arrive for services complaining of problems in distal areas, e.g., carpal tunnel syndrome or plantar fasciitis, our approach is to start at the center and work outward. In fact, many more distal complaints reveal themselves as mere expressions of imbalances at the core, and often resolve without detailed attention to the problem areas as such. Even in cases where there has been a clearly identifiable distal etiology, i.e. a ruptured Achilles tendon, more often than not there is at least some involvement at the core. Limiting attention to a problem area without also addressing related imbalances at the core simply predisposes the body to relapse, no matter how much apparent benefit a client may derive from a given session.

The HSE modus operandi is surprisingly uncomplicated, yet it is anything but random. There are but three basic diagnostic[1] perspectives in somatics, none of which are mutually exclusive of the others. These three are premised on pathological issues of 1) (generally) symmetrical anterior flexion/internal rotation, 2) (generally) symmetrical posterior extension/external rotation, and 3) rotation/tilting that results in postural asymmetry. The first two, flexion/internal rotation and extension/external rotation, are fairly straightforward.

1　The term "diagnosis" is not invoked here in a medical sense, but rather colloquially as a means of analyzing a client's presenting issues so that the somatic educator can proceed in the most appropriate manner.

Asymmetrical rotation, such as occurs when the body tilts or twists, is a bit more involved. Though tilting and twisting appear to involve two separate and distinct planes of motion, in fact, the spine does not so discriminate. Because of the way the vertebrae are designed and assembled, the spine always tilts laterally when it twists, and it always twists when it tilts laterally.[2] Thomas Hanna recognized the propensity of the body to express its neuromuscular problem issues according to these several perspectives and fashioned his approach to undoing the damage wrought by these issues accordingly.

What are All These Lights?

Throughout this text I make intermittent reference to somatic dispositions, such as Red Light reflex, Green Light reflex, or Trauma reflex. I also refer to certain protocols, aka lessons, designed to address these reflex patterns, designated as Lesson 1 for Green Light, Lesson 2 for Trauma, and Lesson 3 for Red Light.[3] These designations are Thomas Hanna's labels for the perspectives discussed above. Among somatic educators it is not unusual to hear these paired terms bandied about interchangeably. When another somatics practitioner tells me that she performed a Lesson 1 with a client, I understand her to mean they had a session for Green Light issues due to that client's patterns of habituation consistent with chronically engaged posterior extensor/ external rotator muscles.

Thomas Hanna did an exemplary job of describing in comprehensive detail exactly what each of these different patterns signified in the human body, as well as how different reflex patterns may interact for an even more convoluted symptomology. In this chapter, I provide only a brief overview of these pathological reflex conditions and of the somatics approach to addressing them. A more detailed discussion of this topic can be found in Thomas Hanna's original text, *Somatics*, which I wholeheartedly recommend.

---

2 I.A. Kapandji, *The Physiology of the Joints, Vol. 3*. Churchill Livingston, 2004.
3 Lessons 1, 2, and 3 each contain elements that address aspects of their counterparts, Red Light, Green Light, and Trauma reflex patterns.

Pathological Reflex Patterns

Thomas Hanna recognized that the effects of sensorimotor amnesia were not random occurrences. Rather, they represented the body's best attempts to adapt to stressors, regardless of whether those stressors were real or imagined. Consequently, somatics is premised on the body's intelligent, and often predictable, response (or reaction) to the world in which it lives. Each individual client has issues rooted in his or her past, contributing to that client's state of being. The clinical somatics protocols developed by Dr. Hanna represent a meticulous approach in addressing any given individual's personal archeology. These protocols offer a framework that takes into account the intelligent design behind a pathological reflex pattern so that somatic educators are able to proceed in their work with clients with the greatest likelihood of successfully resolving clients' issues.

Green Light Posture

Experts note that sixty to eighty percent of adults over the age of forty experience moderate to severe back pain at some point in their lives. The muscles implicated in acute or chronic back pain are invariably involved in the body's Green Light reflex. Green Light reflex, for which we prescribe our Lesson 1, describes a condition in which the body's "Let's go!" muscles—the muscles that propel us forward into action—have become chronically engaged to some degree. This condition is predictably common in industrially developed societies, where timetables, deadlines, and the need or urge to act in a timely fashion define modern culture. The conventional medical profession has an admittedly limited understanding of what causes "nonspecific" back pain, or of how to prevent it or treat it effectively when it does occur. To this day, the specific mechanisms by which back pain is triggered or fails to resolve remains, in many cases, a medical mystery. As you might surmise having read this far, HSE theory offers a plausible explanation and, more importantly, a means of resolution for much of the back pain that people experience.

Back pain is but one guiding symptom of many that can indicate for a Green Light protocol. According to the somatics approach, chronic tightness in the body's posterior muscles, e.g. central extensors of the spine, rhomboids, gluteal muscles, and hamstrings, can be associated with any or all of certain postural features. Green Light features typically include swayback, a tendency toward tight or locked knees or bowleggedness, arms or legs and feet that may appear as externally rotated, and heads that are disproportionately forward in compensation for lumbar lordosis (sway back) or winged scapulae. These imbalances may also produce a predictable assemblage of symptoms, including pinched nerves, herniated discs, sciatica, numbness, headaches, knee problems, tight hamstrings, fatigue, frozen areas, pain in the upper or lower back or in the buttocks, and neck pain. Individuals, e.g., the elderly, who are stuck in pronounced Green Light posture may also be inclined to lurch or fall, as opposed to gliding smoothly as they would if their movements were issued correctly from the center. Hanna noted in his lectures that Green Light propensities are more typically evident in males than females.

Red Light Posture

Red Light reflex entails a chronic activation of the "Whoa!" muscles that stop us, prevent us from going forward, or cause outright retreat. These include many of the larger flexor and internal rotator muscles of the anterior, including the muscles of the abdomen, chest, and legs. These muscles are also associated with the body's withdrawal, or startle reflex, response. Their chronic engagement can often be seen in people who are reticent, anxious, or depressed, or who have had some traumatic experience involving activation of those muscles, e.g., an impending collision. Red Light postures may appear as somewhat hunched or sunken. The knees may appear overly bent or as knock-kneed, this in compensation for the tendency of the buttocks and lower back to protrude rearward, and of the upper body's tendency to generally fold or tilt forward. Meanwhile, the shoulders may be rolled, or even collapsed, inward and the back of the neck compressed as the chin lifts in an ineffectual attempt to adjust for the body's forward tilting.

Problems stemming from Red Light posture typically include shallow breathing, decreased cardiac output and hypertension, depression or anxiety, neck pain, knee problems, frozen parts, and complaints of digestive or sexual function. Women tend more toward Red Light issues than men because, historically, they have more cause for reticence or startle reflex.[4] Elderly persons with Red Light habituation may be prone to a "festinating gait," characterized by small shuffling steps and stumbling to avoid falls due to their center of balance simply being too far forward. Red Light posture calls for a Lesson 3.

In her book, *Train Your Mind Change Your Brain*, Sharon Begley describes watching the Dalai Lama walk on stage, "...with a bit of a stoop, as do many Tibetan monks, shuffling forward with rounded shoulders in a reflexive posture of humility that, over the years, has become his default gait." I mean no disrespect to this eminent man, but I could hardly keep from thinking as I read Begley's account—in her description of His Holiness she provided nothing less than a textbook description of Red Light reflex. I found myself musing whether people inured to a contemplative lifestyle might be predisposed to a predictable assemblage of health issues and an equally predictable trajectory of decline in consequence to however their postures reflect the beliefs and values they hold.[5] It's one thing to cultivate the virtues of introspection and humility. But I see no great benefit if an embodiment of humility, or any other virtue for that matter, culminates in a posture that puts one's health and well-being at risk. Perhaps too much humility is not so good for your body.

---

4 Tom Hanna. *Somatic Exercises*[TM]: *Freeing the Whole Body from Center to Periphery.* CD Lesson 2.
5 Lifestyles and carriage often both reflect and reinforce each other.

Trauma Posture

A third reflex pattern is the Trauma reflex. This pattern is characterized by a body that is tilted to one (or both) sides, or twisted off its symmetrical orientation. Trauma pattern, as you might surmise, is more likely to be caused by injury than by stress, although the stress of some unilateral activities, e.g., the repeated one-sided twisting of a golf swing or of occupational demands such as heavy lifting performed disproportionately from one side, can result, de facto, in a state of injury.

I have often had clients whose obvious need for a Lesson 2 Trauma protocol did seem more a condition, i.e. a reflection on their lifestyle, than the result of any specific identifiable injury. This pattern is also common in mothers accustomed to carrying their toddlers on one hip, as well in those in the habit of slinging heavy burdens across one shoulder, e.g., women with heavy purses, teens laden with book bags, tradesmen with their tools, etc. Even prolonged lounging (listen up, couch potatoes) in an ergonomically incorrect posture can result in Trauma reflex pattern.

Unilateral stressors aside, the body's instinctive reaction to any impending injury is to cringe or flinch from danger as a means of guarding the body. If, having once flinched, the body does not immediately relinquish its initial cringing reaction, an habituated splinting response may ensue, resulting in Trauma posture. Conditions falling under the purview of Trauma protocol can include stiffness or frozen parts, scoliosis, sciatica, headaches, or any of a litany of other complaints involving asymmetry or gait, as well as many issues common to the other reflex patterns mentioned above.

In Sum

None of these deviant postures is mutually exclusive of its counterparts. In fact, we employ the term "dark vice" to describe bodies in advanced stages of simultaneous Green Light/Red Light habituation. Somatic educators frequently see clients whose bodies harbor evidence of two or more of these reflex patterns in combination, the full resolution of which may require a series, albeit usually a short series, of sessions. Part of the role of somatics clinicians is to determine how their clients' bodies may be stuck in various reflex patterns, and to establish a plan, or sequence, of sessions for restoring overall balance in the best way.

Understand that these reflex patterns occur in bodies according to varying degrees. Is it not the case that a person's body or posture must deteriorate to a certain preordained threshold before they can be regarded as a suitable candidate for somatics. Green Light, Red Light, and Trauma reflex designations can describe both varying stages of clear presenting patterns in the body as well as dispositions toward certain patterns that may yet be in their earliest stages. Somatics, therefore, can be entirely appropriate as a preventative measure, even prior to any circumstance in which the need for HSE is clear and compelling.

CHAPTER 4

THE SOMATICS EXPERIENCE

What can you expect from a typical somatics clinical experience? The manner in which different practitioners conduct their clinic varies according to a number of factors, such as the hours they keep for seeing clients, whether they work from home or in an actual clinical setting, whether they have an individual practice or work as part of a group, etc. Some practitioners only teach movement pattern classes, versus seeing clients for clinical sessions. These and other factors will determine their availability and serve to influence whatever first impressions you, as an inquiring client, are inclined to arrive at. I will only speak here regarding my own practice.

Most clients make their initial inquiry over the phone. If time permits, I like to take a few minutes to determine, just superficially, what's prompting someone's inquiry so I have a sense of whether or not somatics may be the best choice for that person. On rare occasions someone's situation will disqualify them outright as a candidate for HSE. I've had relatives inquire on behalf of family members whose mental faculties were severely impaired. Given the collaborative nature of somatics sessions, clients must be able to participate freely, deliberately and consciously.[1] I don't know if any of my colleagues may have customized their approach to work with more compromised populations,[2] but I wouldn't put that beyond the realm of possibility. Now and then someone will call for an appointment and our brief chat will reveal that their physiologic condition makes the likelihood of somatics helping them remote, or that it may be untimely. For example, occasionally, people may be healing

---

1 In seeming contrast to this, Eleanor Criswell-Hanna, Ed.D., has pioneered an application of Hanna Somatics for horses. Please visit www.somaticsed.com/EHS.html to learn more.
2 Some practitioners have reported limited success with dementia patients.

from some acute injury, e.g., a broken limb and I'll put them off until their situation is more resolved.

When clients arrive for a first session, I like to put them at ease while we chat about their circumstance. Quite a few of the folks who end up in my clinic are people who have already been through the mill with other healing or medical modalities, and many feel they've been misunderstood or misguided by other providers. I feel the trust and rapport that ensues from an initial intake is no small consideration. Every client I work with has made a choice to entrust his or her self to my caretaking. This is a responsibility not to be taken lightly.

Getting a sense of somebody's personality can also affect the manner in which a course of sessions unfolds.[3] Though somatic practitioners are adept at reading people's bodies to determine what those bodies need, I find that often-times a client's personality will clue me in to important considerations about their physical state. Bodies usually reflect the psychologies they house, and vice versa. Someone who presents with a personality that is clearly reticent or guarded may be more predisposed to Red Light issues. Your typical Type-A personality tends toward Green Light issues. Yet, in truth, people are rarely that simple.

I'm not prone to psychoanalyzing clients, but the reality is that people can be convoluted; and the more accurate and well rounded a picture one has of a client, the more likely the client's needs can be met in a manner best suited to his or her circumstance. Thomas Hanna noted in his archived lectures, "...this (somatics) work is as much psychological as it is physiological."[4] This important consideration speaks to the impact of somatics on any given individual—how somatics affects both bodies and minds—and also to the regard we somatics practitioners must exercise in fashioning an approach to the clients we work with.

---

3 It is more than mere semantic distinction to say clients enter into a "course of sessions" versus one of "treatment." Somatics practitioners are educators who guide clients in a course of learning. We do not "treat" in the manner of therapeutic modalities.

4 Thomas Hanna's lecture series, July 4, 1990, CD #15. He echoed this sentiment on July 6, 1990, CD #19.

When someone appears to have Red Light issues[5] but is clearly a Type-A personality, I need to file that information away for possible future reference. I may end up addressing their Red Light issues on the table, but then assign home practice movement patterns to them in a way that speaks to their Type-A self to increase the likelihood of compliance.

Returning to the intake procedure, the practitioner wants something of a personal history, though perhaps not the pages and pages that await patients in many medical settings. I like to know, first, what somebody's presenting complaint is, how long it has been going on, its magnitude or effect on the person, the result of any previous attempts to address it, any concomitant issues, any differential factors, e.g., what makes it better or worse, and any identifiable etiology or cause. I also want to determine if there have been any previous insults against the body—falls, surgeries, traumas, etc.—that may have bearing on the current situation. Finally, I like to ask the client what his or her agenda is. What benefits does the client want to see from somatics? Personal agendas vary. Some people want to feel young again, or simply recover from an injury, or resume a cherished activity. Others may just want to regain the dignity and sense of freedom that comes from being able to walk without pain. I can only share in a client's sense of personal vision if I know what it is that the person has in mind.

The Assessment

Once the initial intake is concluded I ask clients to walk about while I observe their gait, and then to stand before me so I can give them a thorough looking over. At my clinic I prefer to have clients stand before a mirror so that I can point out and share with them observations about their posture and carriage. It's quite normal that people will evidence obvious postural imbalances, yet profess total ignorance of them until facing undeniable proof of their condition. Someone who comes in for lower back pain may be oblivious to the fact

---

5 Red Light issues are not generally associated with a "go go go" mindset.

that her head tilts and one shoulder is higher by an inch, or shorter by two, than the other. It's hard to argue with an image in the mirror. Along these lines, I like to shoot a couple digital photos, front and side, as a "before" point of reference. At this stage I'm also making file notes and prioritizing the client's presenting symptoms to determine the best course of action.

Once I've committed myself to starting a client with a particular somatics protocol I ask the client to remove shoes, belts, neckties, pocket items, and jewelry, etc. Clients always remain fully clothed during sessions in somatics; but we don't want restrictive clothing that might impede freedom of movement during the session, or poking holes in our custom-made somatics tables, for that matter. Loose-fitting clothing, e.g., sweats or the like, allows for both comfort and full range of motion. I also ask clients to turn off their cell phones (barring extenuating circumstances) to ensure a distraction-free environment.

I'll usually take this opportunity to explain to the client what all will be entailed with the session, not in great detail, but enough so that the client understands why I'll be moving his or her body or limbs in certain ways to assess range of motion, and what an assisted pandiculation is, and how I will be engaging the client as an active participant in a learning experience. Some clients also take comfort in being assured that pain should never be a part of a session in somatics. For others, e.g., gung-ho types accustomed to deep tissue massage or the like, this may come as something of a disappointment. Depending on how the client is positioned on the table I may also inquire as to their level of comfort: Does the client need a pillow or support anywhere? Does it feel discomfiting to put weight on an injured area? (that sort of thing).

The Session

From here, we proceed into the session. Depending on the protocol opted for, and any considerations particular to the client, sessions typically last anywhere from forty-five–sixty minutes. Notably, and in direct contrast to many massage-type experiences, clinical sessions in somatics are, as a rule, not designed to induce or encourage a deeply relaxed, subcortical state for clients during work in progress. Rather, active cortical participation (attentiveness) is what allows clients to participate fully for best results in restoring voluntary motor control.

Aside from the hands-on aspects, sessions usually conclude with proprioceptive sensing techniques designed to provide clients with the internal resources for self-confirmation of their new and improved postures and abilities.[6] In addition to the protocol itself, sessions also include guidance in specific home practice movement patterns that will serve on an ongoing basis to reinforce the gains achieved during the session. With repeat clients I may take this as an opportunity to review movement patterns assigned from previous sessions to insure that clients are performing them in a correct manner.

As our table work concludes, clients are asked to roll over onto their sides rather than abruptly sitting up prior to standing, as this prevents the undoing of gains that have been made and minimizes the possibility of muscle strain. Once clients are back up on their feet I like to give them a quick body scan, and invite them to stroll about so they can feel for any differences in their bodies. After they've walked a bit, I bring them back to stand in front of the mirror and we scrutinize for changes in their postures generally, as well as at their specific problem areas. Oftentimes, dramatic changes can be observed even beyond the client's presenting issues. In addition, clients often report subjective changes in how they feel after their session.

At this time, if I've taken "before" pictures, I'll follow up with "after" photos for comparison. Photos can be helpful as clients tend to quickly forget (a good thing, I suppose) how their body appeared prior to their somatics experience. Clients not accustomed to self-sensing may not know how to feel or recognize change that has occurred in their own body. Photos can sometimes reveal to them changes they're yet able to feel. In the case of parents who have

---

6 Proprioceptive sensing techniques are designed to progressively narrow any gap between what is perceived subjectively and what is observed objectively.

left their juvenile for a session, the before and after comparisons can provide clear-cut evidence of change, and serve as a compelling incentive to pursue further work as indicated.

Closure

As the session winds down I ask if the client has any questions or comments concerning the work. I always have afterthoughts to share. This closure is important for several reasons. First, the client may actually have questions or comments. Second, this serves as a basis for the somatics experience as an interpersonal process, versus a mere encounter. Third, it speaks to the ongoing nature of the work. I make a point of framing some of my comments in future-speak to emphasize the importance of the continuing and cumulative gains that will result from regular home practice, as well as to reinforce the importance of additional sessions, assuming of course that additional sessions are, in fact, called for.

As a matter of policy I ask new clients to commit themselves to a series of five sessions (this in marked contrast to the open-ended revolving door alluded to previously), to allow for all three protocols, two of which require a separate session for each side of the body. In point of fact some clients require fewer sessions. On occasion, I have discharged clients after a single session because that was all they needed. Even on those rare occasions, clients are encouraged to keep up their home practice patterns as part of their maintenance program.

Before clients walk out the door, I remind them that their body may have undergone quite a lot of change over the last hour or so. Muscles that had previously been engaged 24/7 have now been reeducated to stand down and relax. Drinking plenty of water can help flush toxins such as lactic acid from the body and ease the minor discomforts that sometimes follow a session. I also remind clients that they have, in essence, a new body, and that until they've had twenty-four–forty-eight hours to accustom themselves to their new body they should exercise care in placing old demands on a renewed system, especially in cases where unusual demands for proprioception may be called for. The "unusual demand" category might include dancing, golf, martial arts, skiing, or the like, where the body is expected to perform with unerring balance and precision. Finally, I schedule a follow-up appointment. The ideal interval between somatics sessions is a week or so, though two or three weeks makes for a still manageable approach.

On a final note I encourage clients to contact me in the interim should anything unexpected occur, or if they have questions about their exercise patterns. On occasion, if I have concerns about a client's well-being or about his or her motivation to comply with home practice assignments, I may take the initiative in checking in.

As I mentioned at the beginning of this chapter, the information contained herein is based on the standards of my own practice and serves as no guarantee for how other somatics practitioners conduct their practices. Minor variations notwithstanding, I believe this account captures the essence of a somatics clinical experience.

When to Seek Out HSE

Before proceeding into more detailed discussion of how somatics can work for you, I'd like to touch on another important consideration—namely under what circumstances might you consider yourself a candidate for the somatics method.

I recall one occasion when a client left me a phone message canceling her pending appointment. It wasn't a simple, "I'm sorry, I have to cancel" message. It was one of those rambling messages, the gist of which was that she was feeling much improved as regards her primary health complaint since her last appointment; so she wanted to cancel because she thought she had gotten better; but she wasn't sure she should, and what did I think because she was willing to reschedule if I really thought she should; but she didn't feel it was necessary…and so on. My immediate reaction to her message was that she was being shortsighted in canceling. Granted, in our first session we made good progress, but it had also been evident to me that this woman's body needed more remedial attention than could be afforded by a single session. Of course, I realized also that it was her body, and her prerogative to arrange for her own caretaking as she saw fit. But the prodromal (symptoms in a pre-symptomatic stage) issues in her body, aside from the primary complaint that brought her into my clinic, were sufficiently evident that I was concerned it would only be a matter of time until one or another of them began to express itself at a level of crisis. Clearly, this was a woman who stood to gain substantial benefit by addressing her other issues proactively, rather than waiting for them to become full-blown problems. A little bit of prevention would have gone a long way in her case, as is true of most other people. At the risk of sounding cavalier, I invoke here the old maxim, "Good health doesn't cost; it pays."

Most of the individuals who seek me out for guidance in somatic education do so while in some state of crisis, acute or chronic. More often than not, somatics proves itself an apt resource in addressing a wide range of neuromuscular crisis issues. Yet, I've come to recognize that even given the efficacy of somatics in addressing problems that are already in full bloom, its greatest value lies in prevention and maintenance. I repeat: an ounce of prevention is worth a pound of cure, and HSE represents good value when it comes to prevention. A handful of somatics sessions is a small price to pay for the prospect of a pain-free future.

In Sum

In the words of noted physician and author, Andrew Weil, "Acute and chronic musculoskeletal pain brings more patients to doctors' offices than many other categories of illness combined."[7] Consider for a moment to let the full implication of that statement sink in. Because of its unique emphasis on neu-

---

7 Andrew Weil, M.D., *Spontaneous Healing*. Knopf, 1995.

romuscular intelligence, somatics could single-handedly alleviate much of the burden currently borne by our overwrought healthcare system in preventing or managing complaints of stiffness, inflexibility, pain, and physical decline that so detract from good health and productivity in the twenty-first century. This said, the ideal time for you to engage in a somatics learning experience is before your body submits to its own archeology of insults.

CHAPTER 5

THE PRINCIPLES OF
ASSISTED PANDICULATION

An Overview

Somatics is characterized by a number of indispensable factors, factors which define the work, and without which somatic education would be considerably less effective as a healing and educational modality. Some of these factors, such as the *means whereby*—used in determining a muscle's tonus and range of motion, or *kinetic mirroring*—used to further shorten an already hypertonic muscle, are not unique or original to somatics in and of themselves, but when assembled according to Thomas Hanna's design have uniquely effective ramifications for the human body. One technique, however, stands out in legacy to Hanna's special genius, as an invaluable gift to those who have followed in his path. Assisted pandiculation is the term used to describe the manner in which somatic educators facilitate the release and lengthening of chronically contracted muscles—a sort of "default tonus reset" if you will—without resorting to such invasive measures as forced stretching or even deep tissue massage. Assisted pandiculation is the somatic practitioner's most defining tool in reminding a client's brain how to exercise its own initiative in relaxing tight muscles during any clinical session.

Before delving further into "assisted" pandiculation, let me bring readers up to speed on just what, exactly, it means to pandiculate. Simply put, pandiculation means stretching, but not in the usual manner. "Pan" implies width or breadth (as in panorama), and in old usage "to pandiculate" meant to yawn, and widely at that. The term was once used in a veterinary context to describe stretching such as animals naturally engage in. The *pandicular response* implies stretching such as all animals, including humans, naturally engage in on waking to stimulate the sensory motor cortex. Due to the naturalness of this approach we somatic educators regard pandiculation as substantively different from the kind of agenda-driven stretching people typically engage in.

The usual approach to stretching stems from extrinsic concerns or secondary goals, such as sports and fitness, dancing, gymnastics, or the like—that is, stretching in preparation to get ready for something else. Somatics ascribes to pandiculation as a way to "get ready" for living your life at hand, in other words: stretching (or more correctly lengthening, i.e., relinquishing the hyper part of hypertonus) as a means onto itself. The usual approach to stretching is marginally productive at best, if not downright unhealthy. Aggressive stretching, in particular, does nothing to promote neuromuscular communication, efficiency, or intelligence. Conversely, the somatics pandiculation methods emphasize not only a freer and more flexible you, but the process of self-sensing toward greater neuromuscular control.

In the case of animals, pandiculation is hard wired into their brains—it is instinctive. Imagine a dog or a cat or a mouse waking from a nap. What's the first thing they do? They stretch out their haunches and arch their backs, after which the dog is ready to chase the cat, and the cat is ready to chase the mouse. When was the last time you woke up ready to chase a mouse, or at least willing to indulge yourself the luxury of languorously stretching your body every which way before getting on with your day? Most people's first experience on waking entails fumbling to shut off their alarm clock before jumping out of bed to slurp down a cup of coffee and a fat laden donut or a bowl of sugary cereal as they rush off to start their day. Talk about insults! People should be so smart as to take a cue from their pets and make somatically correct stretching a priority on waking.

In somatics we utilize two different kinds of pandiculations, those performed by oneself for oneself (self-pandiculations—to be addressed a little later on), and those in which one person (preferably a trained professional) assists another person. Somatic educators are thoroughly trained in both these methods. You might be wondering at this point, if self-stretching works so well for the cat, why would you need someone's assistance to help you pandiculate? The reasons for assisted pandiculations will become evident as you read on.

Assisted Pandiculation

Assisted pandiculation maneuvers are akin to Taijiquan's Push Hands practices in representing the very embodiment of softness and harmony between two engaging forces. I recall making that same association with pushing hands during my first day in class as a Hanna somatics trainee, when I and my fellow students were introduced to the theory and practice nuances of the assisted pandiculation technique.

During any assisted pandiculation of someone else's muscle it is essential to find and use just the correct amount of force—no more and no less—to orchestrate an isotonic state in which a subsequent *controlled release* of muscle tonus provides an optimum of sensorimotor feedback to the brain. In this manner somatic educators can facilitate the disarmament of a muscle's natural tendency to resist yielding up its tightness, in favor of helping it to achieve its full potential for relaxation and length, as well as its responsiveness both to and for neural impulses.

It is in calling the brain to task through assisted pandiculations that one of the primary roles of the cerebral cortex—as a reviewer and inhibitor of emotions and reflex patterns stemming from the middle and lower brain regions—can be implemented to check and recalibrate errant reflex patterns that serve as a template for hypertonic musculature.

How is it that HSE practitioners are able to exercise a quality of sensitivity in working with clients to achieve these results? Two skills, (which are mutually reinforcing) come immediately to mind. First is the aforementioned Tin Jing-like listening skill, ala Tai Chi's Pushing Hands, which I discussed in

Chapter 2. HSE practitioner trainees typically develop the sensitivity necessary for this skill as one part of their training. Second, in a manner somewhat analogous to what is known in psychology as the Theory of Mind,[1] somatic educators must be skilled at an equivalent Theory of Mind AND Body. This ability is what enables us to discern not only the state of a client's body at any given moment during clinical work, but also its likely response, and our attuned response to its response, during assisted pandiculations. The same Theory of Mind and Body applies during spoken directions in the case of guided self-pandiculation patterns. Both of these skills likely involve unconscious reliance on mirror neurons as practitioners seek to align with the internal states of their clients.[2] These two skills, among others, enable HSE practitioners to work with clients in tacit collaboration for best results.

Assisted pandiculation, as a technique, is brilliant in both its simplicity and its effectiveness in overriding the tendency toward entrenchment, so that chronically engaged muscles more freely loosen their grips on themselves. Addressing chronic muscular tonus at its source, in the brain, versus at its point or area of expression in the muscles, is the only effective way to achieve lasting improvement. Barring assisted pandiculation, the likelihood is that muscles stuck in varying degrees of contraction will continue to aggravate their condition by becoming increasingly more stuck over time rather than looser. This is why persons who try to force-stretch tight muscles achieve temporary flexibility or relief only. The gradual exacerbation of tight muscles is also exactly how our aforementioned "archeology of insults" degenerates the body, eroding its flexibility and its ability over time to self-sense. Degeneration such as this stems from the accumulation of tension and its entrenchment into habituated patterns, which is the very opposite of dissipation and the release of tension toward a fuller freedom of movement.

---

1 The "Theory of Mind" describes one's ability to extend awareness beyond his or her own limited first-person perspective to reasonably anticipate (from) another's thought or feeling process. You do this unconsciously anytime you finish someone's sentence for them or consider another's point of view.

2 Daniel J. Siegal, *The Mindful Therapist.* Norton, 2010.

Muscle Minutia

Without delving too deeply here into the finer points of alpha-gamma motor neuron coactivation and intrafusal and extrafusal muscle fibers (of unlikely interest to lay readers in any case) I will foray into a brief technical aside. In point of fact, muscles do not become increasingly tighter over time, however much that may feel to be the case, at least not in quite the way we commonly assume they do. Rather than an entire muscle becoming tighter, what occurs more precisely, is that greater numbers of muscle fibers in a given muscle become, and remain, chronically engaged. Individual muscle fibers are assembled into bundles of motor units. Muscles engage incrementally during normal use, so that only as many of these motor units as necessary for a given task are activated. The motor units that do engage, do so fully. This is known as the All-or-None Principle in which all the muscle fibers comprising any given motor unit either contract completely or not at all. Thus, some motor units engage fully while others, held in reserve, may not engage at all. If the demands on a muscle for a given action increase, additional reserve motor units engage, also fully, to handle the extra demand. Thus, it is not the case that already-engaged motor units engage more fully. Muscle motor units are either turned on or off, there's no middle ground. Individual muscles may contain hundreds of motor units.[3] Motor units, themselves, depending on the size and role of the muscle in question, can contain anywhere from five to two thousand individual muscle fibers.[4] This explains how sensorimotor amnesia can also occur incrementally, in just part of a muscle, and compound over time as additional fibers and motor units in that muscle may be recruited into chronic engagement. In this manner, there is quite literally the potential for an archeology of engagement, according to how muscle fibers and motor units are called into play.

This also explains why pain or injury, or the effects of sensorimotor am-

---

3 Joseph Hamill and Kathleen M. Knutzen, *Biomechanical Basis of Human Movement*. Lippincott, Williams & Wilkins, 2006.
4 Bill Garoutte, Ph.D., M.D., *Survey of Functional Anatomy*. Jones Medical Pub., 1981.

nesia, can be localized to parts of a muscle only, without seeming to affect the entire length or span of that muscle. And it explains why muscles can remain functional, to a degree, even when they've incurred some level of injury or SMA. It may be possible to rely on a muscle that has been damaged, or is amnesiac, yet only feel pain or restriction in that muscle at the point where the damaged or amnesiac area is called on to perform.

Infrastructural Decline

Another way to visualize the body's tendency toward progressive sensorimotor decline is to frame that decline in terms of a hypothetical driving scenario. Imagine a new stretch of roadway running between two adjacent cities. That road, in perfect repair, is like a healthy muscle with its traffic flowing freely. However, if some situation occurs that causes a specific location along that stretch of road to develop serious potholes, the flow of commuter traffic becomes impeded. The usually fast-moving traffic must now slow nearly to a halt to navigate past. Once past the slowdown, normal traffic flow resumes. But over time the usual demands of traffic traversing this road along its potholed stretch create a tendency to logjam that cannot improve until the road is repaired. In fact, the situation can only get worse, not better, if steps are not taken to repair the infrastructure. Now imagine that the erratic traffic flow causes new potholes to appear not far from the original problem, and that their effect on traffic flow compounds the problem. The entire remaining length of highway may still be in good repair; but the potholes, though local in their immediate effect, serve to reduce the ease and efficiency of the overall driving experience. Furthermore, the prospect of additional future potholes will only continue to aggravate driving conditions, until eventually a once-pleasant drive becomes one fraught with frustration and inconvenience, perhaps even accidents. This is not at all unlike the scenario of a muscle (or a body) that becomes chronically engaged, first in one small place, due perhaps to just a minor pothole-like insult, only to have its vulnerability for further and more complicated decline heightened as additional insults are added into the mix.

As long as we're on the road here, let's remember that potholes don't fix themselves. First, there's a causative event, something (an insult) that results in a pothole. Then someone has to notice or experience the consequence of the pothole (e.g., subjective pain, or observation by a third party). Then someone has to report (afferent messages) that there's a problem. Once a report has been filed and processed, word has to come down from the central highway office (the brain) in order for a maintenance crew to be sent (efferent messages) to the scene to enact repairs (via somatics) so that smooth traffic flow (differentiation and control) can resume. Keep in mind, though, that any and all repairs are entirely contingent on the problem being reported in the first place. If no problem is perceived, say because drivers are distracted on their cell phones (due to SMA), no repair is likely to be forthcoming. Finally, the repair of any given pothole can't guarantee against future potholes. Ongoing infrastructural oversight (home practice movement patterns) is a must.

Assisted Pandiculation is Collaborative

Unlike many therapeutic experiences, in which something may be done to, at, or on the body, assisted pandiculation is designed as an educational experience requiring a collaborative effort between client and provider. No somatic practitioner can effectively assist in the pandiculation of your muscles absenting your conscious and willing participation. If the deliberate attention and intention of your brain is omitted from the equation, the desired results will not ensue.

> Attention and intention on your part as a somatics client are necessary components because they represent the involvement of the cortical brain. It is in the brain, not in the muscles themselves, where the template for errant sensorimotor circuits must be recalibrated.

In order to correct the errant pattern in any durable fashion, the new correct pattern must first be experienced in the voluntary cortex before it can be relegated, through reinforcement (repeated practice) to a more permanent status in the subcortex where all such patterns are destined for storage.

How Can You Participate for Best Results?

Given the collaborative nature of the work, it follows that best results can be obtained when both parties contribute in the best way to the process of change. How, then, can you best participate as a collaborative "pandiculee" to enhance your own healing process?

Unfortunately, the same issues of sensorimotor amnesia that serve as a basis for someone's seeking bodily change can undermine their optimally effective participation and contribution. The more seriously compromised your self-sensing ability, the less able you may be to exercise precise control of your muscles during any given assisted pandiculation, at least until you are taught how to do so. Hypothetically, if you already had perfect self-sensing abilities throughout your body, you might disqualify yourself as a candidate for somatic education. Why fix it if it ain't broke? However, as the old saying implies, nobody's perfect. It's a rare person who hasn't forfeited their ability for self-sensing somehow somewhere in their body—it's just part of being human. Not to worry though, as somatic educators are well prepared to deal with this eventuality. In fact, it is the essence of our job to help you (re)learn how to self-sense. That's the E (education) in H.S.E.

Even if you suffer from fairly extensive SMA, you may expedite your learning process by anticipating certain considerations. Generally, in any case where the ability of the brain to communicate with the muscles has been compromised, auxiliary measures will have been activated. The brain and body are very good at compensating. This human ability to compensate, or adapt, represents an evolutionary Plan B for staying alive—for surviving— but not necessarily for surviving in the most intelligent and sustainable way.

In fact, it is the very propensity of the brain and body for counterproductive compensatory measures that provides a basis for this field.

One general skill that you will certainly find to be of inestimable value in obtaining best results from your somatics experience is motor planning. Motor planning can substantially enhance your grasp of many of the other qualities mentioned in Chapter 2, including methodical and differentiated movement, proprioception, "listening" to your body, and sustainability. In its simplest guise, motor planning is the process of forming a mental representation, or a mental rehearsal, of how your body will enact a given behavior, such as an assisted or self-pandiculation, *prior to actually doing so*, and then hovering briefly just at that boundary between intention and action. When you (only) imagine enacting a movement, just to a point of almost doing it, the planning process will evoke the beginnings of a somatic, or motor, response. Once you become adept at motor planning you'll be amazed at how much happens with your internal mechanisms during the lead-up stage to an actual execution of any overt muscular action.

Common sense suggests that you'll learn a desired skill faster and better by rehearsing it. In his book, *Outliers: the Story of Success*, Malcolm Gladwell stipulates ten thousand hours of practice at any given task as requisite to achieving "mastery."[5] I can assure you that you won't need anywhere near ten thousand hours of practice at somatics before gaining satisfactory results. That said, there is a neurological basis for the maxim, "practice makes perfect," as continued actual rehearsal of motor events is known to result in long-term synaptic potentiation (LTSP), meaning the efficiency of synaptic activity between neurons becomes streamlined to a given task with repeated firings.

Even mental rehearsal can produce measurable change. To cite one example of an oft repeated experiment, Alvaro Pascual-Leone M.D., Ph.D., confirmed the value of mental rehearsal of a motor activity by demonstrating that piano students engaging in mental practice alone produced the same changes

---

5 Malcolm Gladwell, *Outliers: the Story of Success*. Little Brown, 2008.

in their motor systems as students engaged at actual practice.[6] However, there is a more profound neurological mechanism involved here that goes beyond the effects of mere practice. In 1985, Swedish psychiatrist and neuroscientist, David Ingvar, coined the term and seeming non sequitur, "memory of the future,"[7] to describe how our past experiences contribute to whatever expectations we hold for our future. Motor planning (not perfunctory planning, mind you, but planning that is profoundly deliberate) is essentially the forming of a memory of the future. By imagining, or anticipating, and almost implementing movements with your body—which, in the case of somatic pandiculations constitute a very specialized type of movement, performed perhaps at a level of nuance—prior to enacting these movements, your brain forms a memory of that which has been imagined before having had the actual full experience. More recently, Daniel Siegel described a process whereby interoception facilitates a more "distanced" metarepresentation of the body for enhanced regulatory oversight of conscious processes.[8] Thus are the seeds of change planted, simply via the motor planning, prior to enacting assisted or self-pandiculations.

> Given that it is usually easier to practice and refine a skill you've already had some experience at, as opposed to learning that skill from scratch, motor planning makes for an effective learning device in that it allows you to more efficiently organize your body and its behavior during motor tasks. Motor planning infuses a "fine motor" quality into gross motor tasks and renders already-fine motor tasks "finer."

A similar dynamic, albeit with a different explanation and label, is offered in *Job's Body*[9] by Dean Juhan in his description of what he calls "sensory en-

---

6 Doidge, *The Brain*.
7 Goldberg, *The Executive Brain*.
8 Siegal, *The Mindful Therapist*.
9 Juhan, *Job's Body*.

grams." We've already seen how imagining a motor activity stimulates motor neurons, providing a subtle quality of sensory feedback even without blatant motor involvement. According to Juhan, rehearsal of an event results in the formation of a template of sorts, allowing repetition of the event to proceed with increased, even automatic, efficiency as the sensory memory of that event effectively comes to control its motor expression. Event rehearsal causes the synaptic connections between neurons to become increasingly efficient at processing information associated with that event.

Motor planning, as such, calls into play aspects of the brain's frontal lobes, particularly the motor and pre-motor cortex, which are responsible for, among other tasks, planning and anticipation of consequences for one's behavior,[10] as well as the left supramarginal gyrus located in the parietal lobe, required for the conjuring up of intended motor actions prior to execution,[11] and the anterior insula and anterior cingulate.[12] In fact, there is a growing body of evidence to suggest that mere thinking necessarily entails some level of doing, and that the very act of thinking does itself activate motor neurons, without any conscious intention to act.[13] Motor planning as an acquired skill can enable you to derive a greater and more direct benefit from your HSE experience.

In sum, there is an inverse correlation between people's ability to recognize sensorimotor amnesia in their own body and the extent of that amnesia. The more SMA you have the less able you may be to be consciously aware of it. When working with clients in my clinical practice I regularly elicit feedback during sessions, e.g., How does this feel? or, How does that compare? The more compromised a client's body is, the more likely the client will report, "I can't tell," or, "I don't feel anything." Sensorimotor amnesia, by

---

10 Goldberg, *The Executive Brain*.

11 V.S. Ramachandran, *A Brief Tour of Human Consciousness*. Pi Press, 2004.

12 Siegal, *The Mindful Therapist*.

13 This according to multiple separate sources first cited by Thomas Hanna in, *The Body of Life*, 1979, including; neurophysiologists Roger W. Sperry, and Edmund Jacobson, and Roland C. Davis, and F.J. McGuigan, and Robert Malmo, and the research team of Smith, Brown, Toman and Goodman. The same is subsequently cited, as well, in *The Brain That Changes Itself*, by Norman Doidge. Thomas Metzinger echos this sentiment in, *The Ego Tunnel*, 2009.

definition, implies a compromised ability to self-sense. So, if you do recognize that you have sensorimotor amnesia, and you do elect to seek out a qualified somatics practitioner to help you restore full sensorimotor function, try to keep an open mind during your learning experience. Self-sensing is a learned skill that may take time and considerable practice to master.

The great majority of somatics exercises involve movements that are small and subtle, often so understated as to render them (initially) challenging for many people. That such a sweeping element of challenge exists at all serves as sad commentary that a loss of precise muscular control leaves so many people unable to experience their own bodies except via movements that are large and exaggerated. Often, these same folks are hardest pressed to develop an appreciation for the real value of movements that are small and precise.

Your chosen practitioner will probably ask you to engage in movements that challenge your ability for precise muscular control. These movements will not entail undue exertion, or push you to exceed your physical limits in any way. Nor should they cause pain. In fact, what you'll likely find most challenging are the nuanced features of the movement. You will be asked to make your best attempt to control your movements slowly and precisely without outright physical exertion. It bears repeating that this will require both practice and patience on your part.

A Typical Course of Sessions

Consider the experience of a hypothetical client. Imagine a scenario in which someone (let's call him Joe) spends three months on crutches while recuperating from a broken leg. Before breaking his left leg, Joe worked as an appliance technician, often lifting heavy parts and working with his body engaged in awkward positions. After the recuperative period Joe's cast comes off; the crutches are cast aside, and his life resumes. In the interim, the muscles of Joe's damaged leg have atrophied. Just as the muscles in his injured leg have weakened, the muscles of his uninjured leg have endured an added workload from carrying his body around on crutches all day long and favoring the injured leg. As a result, these muscles have become stronger. In fact, it's not only the muscles of Joe's legs that have been affected by the injury and recovery process. Many other muscles throughout his body have been affected as well as they've striven for some sense of equilibrium during the recovery process. While on crutches Joe's torso on the injured left side, extending from his hip up along through his ribs, has splinted into a tight contraction due to his unconscious favoring of that side while gimping around in such an unnatural manner. Simultaneously, Joe developed asymmetrical tightness in his upper back muscles and throughout the axillary (armpit) area on both sides of his body from weighting himself on his crutches.

After Joe's body has adopted all these compensatory measures to manage and protect itself during its healing process, how can these muscles possibly be expected to simply give up their day job? Nobody likes being fired or downsized, and the muscles in Joe's body are no exception. Once Joe's femur has healed his body must deal with a whole new slew of readjustments and compensations. Depending on how resilient and intelligent his body is, and depending on what the resumption of normal demands entails, the likelihood remains that some of the compensatory measures will linger as new, albeit errant, patterns in Joe's body. He walks with a pesky limp that subsides somewhat, but not completely, as his injured leg rebuilds its strength. Along with the aforementioned lower body problems, there is now the issue of compensatory tightness incurred in his shoulders, upper back, chest, neck, and abdomen from supporting himself on those crutches. In short, Joe's fractured leg has healed, but the rest of his body is a mess as a result of that one major insult [Figures 5-1a & b].

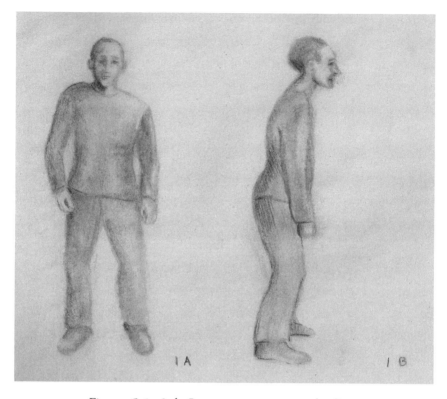

Figures 5-1a & b. Joe, post-trauma, post-healing.

After a few months, Joe no longer notices that he still limps. His friends have stopped noticing as well. All parties have become "habituated" to Joe's carriage and movement. His broken leg is but a thing of the past. However, Joe hasn't been sleeping as well as he did before his injury and his back is now giving him problems—it feels "tense and tight." He notices his libido is diminished and this has caused some stress in his marriage. As the advice offered by his conventional medical provider hasn't proven particularly helpful, Joe decides it's time to explore for non-conventional help. A friend recommends a bodywork professional, a therapist who cleverly observes during their first session that Joe's shoes are not wearing evenly and shows Joe that one of his legs—the left one—is shorter than the other (must've occurred when he broke his leg). Joe is advised to get orthotic shoe inserts to equalize his legs. The orthotics feel okay at first, but they don't stop Joe from limping and they do not alleviate his back pain, which has become worse. Joe consults another health professional. And then another. After a series of failed attempts at recovering the state of health he enjoyed before his broken leg, Joe finds me—or any other somatic educator.

I look Joe over and conclude that, indeed, he is a mess, but not beyond redemption. Joe is evidencing the effects of Trauma and Green Light habituation, as well as Red Light issues. As I chat with Joe, taking his history and developing a sense of him, I surmise that the Trauma symptoms (so noted because of his postural asymmetry) are likely due to the broken leg. I also note that his Red Light symptoms (evidenced by his shoulders and chest curled forward in flexion) are not especially pronounced and that, curiously, they hardly seem characteristic of his overall personality or indicative of his lifestyle. Perhaps they're just a holdover from three months of hovering over crutches. Joe's Green Light symptoms (surmised from his over-arched lower back and forward-jutting head), on the other hand, seem more "him." My impression in this regard is reinforced by Joe's assertiveness in presenting his case. I decide to start by addressing Joe's most pressing issues, the trauma stemming from his leg injury. Before I begin working with Joe I share my thoughts regarding his situation and explain to him how his somatics experience is likely to unfold. I emphasize that the results from any individual session may vary and that he will most certainly require at least several sessions to comprehensively address all his issues.

On the Table—Joe's Dimmer Switch

Prior to beginning our table work I explain to Joe what an assisted pandiculation is and how it works. Starting out with a maneuver designed to help Joe restore full function to his latissimus dorsi muscle, which I suspect is implicated in his back pain and sleeplessness, I ask Joe to contract this muscle gradually but firmly prior to his releasing it very slowly. Instead, Joe puts the full force of his waist and shoulder into yanking his arm and back taut, as if he were fighting against me. This reveals something about the extent of Joe's sensorimotor amnesia and prompts me to adjust my approach.

My new first order of business becomes teaching Joe how to sense this muscle. We accomplish this by shelving, for the time being, the assisted pandiculation for the "lat" muscle. Instead, I ask Joe to pay close attention while I palpate this muscle and its structural attachments, modeling for him its role in his body so that he can begin to feel its differentiated function. This will enable him to slowly assume initiative in enacting for himself the movements I have modeled for him. This approach is known in somatics terminology as the "means whereby." I ask Joe to contract his latissimus muscle at varying levels of engagement, before releasing it slowly, bit by bit, to improve his differentiation. Once Joe has accomplished a more refined sense of how to contract just this muscle we can go back to the assisted pandiculation with a greater likelihood of his muscles not working at odds with each other. Now, as Joe contracts his latissimus muscle, I ask him again to release it very slowly. At first, Joe's ability to control this muscle is still all or nothing, with little middle ground. Granted, he is better able after being coached to confine his contraction to just the muscle on which we are focusing (so we're headed in the right direction), but his activation of it reminds me of a light switch that offers only on or off options. After some coaxing and a few more attempts, Joe arrives at a point where he is able to demonstrate improved control by utilizing the "dimmer switch"[14] strategy. He is becoming better able to isolate and release just this muscle from its contracted state in a more gradual fashion, as if he were adjusting a lamp by slowly turning down its dimmer switch.

After just a few rehearsals there remain only localized lapses in control.

---

14   Individuals with poorly developed or compromised muscle functions often compensate for their lack of precise control by conscripting synergists (muscles that perform a similar task) in lieu of the targeted muscle. As a result, the activation of the targeted muscle is poorly differentiated. Clients can avoid this tendency to over-engage muscles during contraction by contracting the targeted muscle slowly, as if they were adjusting up a dimmer switch. The same strategy, in reverse, allows for a precisely controlled *release* of tension, and a more effective relinquishment of SMA.

Reminiscent of the potholes alluded to earlier in this chapter, these lapses pinpoint the epicenters associated with Joe's sensorimotor amnesia. In fairly short order Joe has begun to release the chronic tension from his back and has gained an increase in the latissimus muscle's range of motion by some several inches. With the release of tension he has also achieved an obvious improvement in the suppleness of his upper back, and an improved ability to differentiate these same muscles. Joe's brain has begun to reprioritize its awareness of this part of his body.

As our session continues we gradually work our way around Joe's body. When we get to his legs he reminds me that one leg is shorter than the other. I confirm that, indeed, his left leg does appear shorter. After two assisted leg pandiculations, both Joe's legs measure at equal length and it occurs to him that he'll no longer be needing the orthotic shoe inserts he's been wearing since seeing that first therapist. In fact, dispensing with those now unnecessary inserts will help to ensure that they don't offset or undo the gains he has made in this session.

Our first session over, Joe is noticeably straighter when viewed from the side. Frontally, as he stands before the mirror, Joe's body seems almost over-compensated now to his right [Figures 5-2a & b]. I assure him this is nothing to be concerned about for the time being, as his body may well right itself before our next scheduled session. Notably, and without his orthotics, Joe seems to have lost his limp. Before he leaves, I advise him how he might use what he observes in a mirror to further improve his self-sensing abilities at home. I also give Joe instructions on how to integrate somatic movement patterns specific to his situation into a daily home practice routine to continually reinforce the new freedom his body and brain have gained. This follow-up homework is mandatory, not optional, if he wishes to maintain his improvements. Joe is on his own until our next visit.

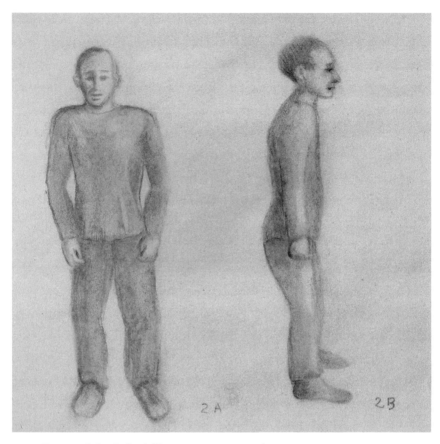

Figures 5-2a & b. A Trauma session results in some improvement.

When Joe returns for a next session two weeks later he looks quite different from his initial arrival. He reports improved energy (...didn't even know my energy had fallen off since that injury), and better sleeping. Also, friends and family have commented on "something being different" about him. I opt for a Red Light lesson for his second session. He needs a Green Light session, but I want to first resolve his Red Light issues, anticipating that he may gain greater benefit from a Green Light session if we get his Red Light "stuff" out of the way first. After his Red Light session Joe stands more erect, and even appears more youthful in his carriage. He continues with his designated home practice exercises, including some new patterns, over the next two weeks.

When Joe comes back for a third, Green Light, session he reveals that it is more than just his posture that is now erect. The Red Light lesson seems to have alleviated the chronic low-grade stress in his abdomen, allowing for improved circulation and a return of his libido. I guide Joe in a Green Light session and the results, though noticeable, are in his particular case and by comparison to his earlier changes, less dramatic. I recognize and explain to Joe that we are now addressing some of his more deeply seated issues, older stuff that was there in his body well prior to his broken leg, and that one or two additional sessions may be necessary to comprehensively resolve his remaining issues. After this lesson Joe is visibly improved in his carriage, yet he opts to discontinue his sessions. As far as he's concerned he got what he came for and simply is not committed to doing the work necessary beyond that which provided a certain immediate level of gratification. Had Joe stayed on for one or two additional sessions he would certainly have made additional headway in relinquishing residual sensorimotor issues. As it stands, the level at which Joe has set his personal bar for himself—namely just at pre-trauma level—has been achieved, and then some. By my reckoning he still has quite a bit of room for improvement. Unfortunately, Joe has made the decision to reconcile himself to living with (what I see as) still unresolved issues. There is every possibility, indeed every probability, that these remaining issues will resurface at some future point in more dramatic fashion. Or, Joe may hold these issues in abeyance and perhaps even make some progress on his own, if he keeps up diligently with his home practice movement patterns. Overall, Joe's account is fairly typical, if there is such a thing.

Wherever possible, we somatic educators make our best effort to encourage clients to explore for the best state of physical health they can possibly achieve. In Joe's case an assortment of pandiculation techniques (assisted and self), along with other somatics measures, were employed to alleviate the far-reaching effects of his one injury. Imagine if Joe resorted instead to a life of orthotics, painkillers, and Viagra, masking over his symptoms in lieu of addressing their underlying causes. Surely, his health and well-being would have continued along a downward trajectory, culminating in a much deteriorated posture and quality of life. As it turned out, Joe ended up much better off than he'd been prior to his somatics experience, but he could have achieved even more progress had he stuck it out with additional sessions [Figures 5-3a & b, 5-4a & b]. As somatics educators, our interest extends beyond the mere resolution of existing problems. Ideally, we want teach clients how to avoid future problems by adopting a somatic mindset.

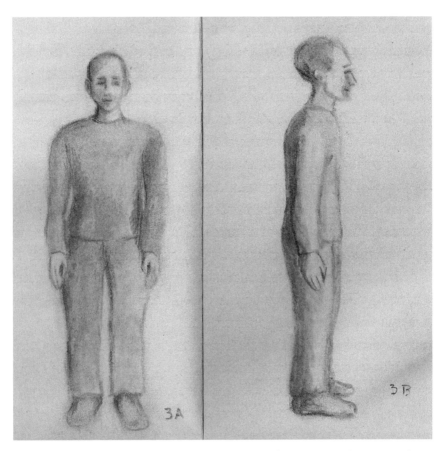

Figure 5-3a & b. The "Possible" Joe, not perfect, but much improved.

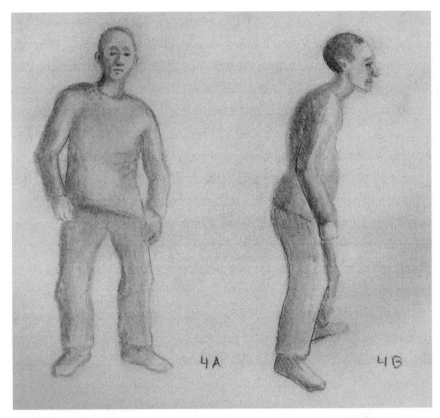

Figure 5-4a & b. The "Worst Scenario" Joe, sans HSE.

Joe's case was a purely fictional account designed to give readers some insight into the way Hanna's assisted and self-pandiculation techniques can be employed to undo the effects of sensorimotor amnesia and restore full and healthy functioning to the body's sensorimotor system. Every client is unique, and it is the role of the somatics practitioner to adjust his or her clinical approach to the particular needs of any individual client.

Notably, our fictional client's premature departure reflects many a real client who may be either impatient for results, shortsighted in his or her unwillingness to commit for sustainable and lasting gain, or penny-wise and pound-foolish in anticipating the long-term value of a short series of four–six sessions. I suspect this can be attributed to a certain unfortunate enculturation that has most folks setting their own personal best bar for health and wellness far below the limits of their true potential.

Significant improvement from somatics is often, but not always, quite rapid, and lasting gain does require an ongoing commitment to regular practice on one's own. As for the expenditures involved, the initial costs associated with somatic sessions are sometimes a bit higher in comparison to other body/ mind therapies, but compare very favorably over the long term when weighing actual results against the number of sessions necessary. Savvy consumers will consider that somatics is an investment in the future—one that will continue to pay very generous dividends for as long as you choose to reap them.

Self-Pandiculation

The principles of pandiculation can also be employed in a non-collaborative manner. Individuals practicing on their own can utilize a controlled release, either in disengaging contracted muscles slowly on their own, or in releasing muscular effort slowly to the force of gravity. This is a fundamental aspect of many of the somatic movement patterns such as were prescribed to our client Joe for home practice. Of course, the pandiculation methods we teach clients are carefully selected and tailored according to the client's particular needs.

Note that many HSE movement patterns can easily be mistaken (tip of the iceberg fallacy) by casual observers not schooled in somatic nuance as to be indistinct from ordinary stretching exercises. Ordinary stretching, as such, is primarily a physiologic event, devoid of the focused attention that characterizes optimal learning experiences. What renders somatics patterns so effectively distinct from ordinary stretching is the "intra" aspect, i.e., the motor planning, as well as the overall emphasis on self-sensing, so that the experience one has is every bit as cortical as it is physiologic.

Thomas Hanna noted in his teachings that an additional (sixth) sense ought to be recognized, and accorded primacy even over the usual five. The sense he had in mind was that of self-sensing, or sensorial awareness, aka interoception, so that people everywhere could learn to discern and monitor their own internal state and condition. Indeed, many of my clients who also happen to be fitness enthusiasts marvel at the level of focused attention required to execute somatics maneuvers in a fashion that is both correct and beneficial.

Remember that the movement patterns themselves are only effective in redressing sensorimotor amnesia in accordance with the conscious attention and intention of the person practicing them. Another example of brain research supporting this contention: Michael Merzenich, Ph.D., a leading researcher on brain plasticity, performed numerous experiments, albeit with primates, which led him to conclude that rehearsal of tasks in an automatic manner was sufficient to alter brain maps, but not in any durable fashion. Lasting change, Merzenich found, occurred only when his test subjects were inspired to pay close attention to whatever task was at hand.[15] Similarly, even though you may be going through the motions of HSE patterns, the full effects of an otherwise well-indicated pandiculation will fall short of best results without your focused attention. Therefore, you should always make your best effort to be fully present to yourself to gain optimal benefit.

---

15 Doidge, *The Brain.*

CHAPTER 6

THE LIMITS OF SOMATIC EDUCATION

Given my enthusiasm on the topic, readers may form the impression that I regard somatics as a panacea. Nothing could be further from the truth. Somatics is quite useful as far as it goes, which is saying a lot; but it is hardly a cure-all for all of mankind's ills.

Somatics is a neuromuscular reeducation tool and, as such, is useful to the extent that some malfunction as expressed in the motor component of the neuromuscular system is implicated due to sensorimotor amnesia. But that's it. Somatics cannot correct conditions of nerve degradation. Nor does it claim to correct problems with the body that have a basis in structural faults or defects, or in system faults not having to do with motor issues. Somatics will not act directly to undo or reverse the effects of poor dietary habits, the ravages of free radicals, or the aging effects of hormonal decline, etc. Somatics will do nothing to stop hair loss.

That said, many of the body's systems are interrelated and interdependent. The effects of stress on any system are certain to have some effect on other systems. Often, problems with the nervous system or with the body's structural aspects will have muscular issues that are concomitant—the same could be said for the digestive system or the endocrine system—and concomitant issues such as these may be addressed by somatics.

The very first client I had the privilege of working with (referenced briefly in Chapter 1) was a woman who had suffered a severe stroke, resulting in paralysis to the left side of her body. She contacted me by phone to ask if I might do something to relieve the chronic tightness in her left hand. As one result of her stroke, which occurred several years prior, her hand went into spasm and simply stayed that way, balled up into a tight fist. She'd had no improvement since her stroke despite repeated consultations with her physician, her acupuncturist, and her physical therapist. At the time of our first consultation I wondered if maybe I'd bitten off more than I should chew. How could it be possible that I might have something of genuine value to offer this woman where other, more-learned minds, had been unable to provide relief? Nevertheless, I decided to make my best effort to help this woman.

A cursory examination revealed that she'd lost probably ninety-nine percent of her ability to voluntarily control the muscles of her hand. Even given this loss, the corollary was that she retained one percent or so of her voluntary control, and that modicum of control, as it turned out, was all we needed to effect dramatic change, to induce the chronically contacted flexor muscles of her left hand to release their grip. We were just five minutes into our first session when her left hand opened easily and completely in response to an assisted pandiculation. She was immediately in tears and I was frankly humbled. Mind you, she was my first ever client. Unfortunately, her progress was limited to that one major advance. Despite repeated follow-up sessions the drama appeared to have played itself out in that first five minutes. She did not regain voluntary control of the muscles of her left hand and was only able to open it by using her right hand to do so, a fact that hardly mitigated her delight in doing so on a regular basis. Regrettably, the nerve damage from her stroke appeared too extensive to allow for more global improvement, though she and I continued to meet periodically in hopes of further improvement. The muscle tonus that kept her hand balled up in a tight fist was merely concomitant to the nerve damage; and, happily, that tonus was the sort of problem issue that somatics could address. However, the more global limitations of her nerve damage seemed beyond the reaches of somatic education.[1]

---

1 However, some four years subsequent to our initial session, this client was able to move her left leg, raising and lowering it and maneuvering it about from side to side, along with some ability to dorsiflex her foot. She can stand and walk with the assistance of a cane and a foot brace. I attribute much of her continuing improvement to somatics as she eschewed other therapies (or, rather, was eschewed by them when her insurance ran out) in favor of HSE.

Frequently, structural or nervous system conditions, as well as systemic issues that have become cyclical and self-reinforcing, will cause complications with the body's musculature. Sometimes these muscular complications can, in turn, compound their own underlying causes, or lead to other seemingly unrelated problems. Any or all of these complications can obfuscate a clear picture of cause and effect. In a case where muscular tightness causes nerve problems (e.g., pain or numbness such as occurs when chronically tight muscles pinch nerves in the lower back to cause sciatica), addressing the tightness in the muscles will likely provide a measure of relief to the nerves. However, if the sciatica is due to a vertebral subluxation (a structural problem), the structural fault must be corrected first before any neuromuscular work is likely to have lasting effect. In some such cases, somatics may facilitate the necessary structural realignment, although we make no claims to that effect.

In other cases, chiropractic (or whatever modality accomplishes the job) may be more direct in paving the way prior to attention to the errant muscular patterns. The same rationale suggests that non-structural issues such as adhesions and scar tissue might be best dealt with by massage-type modalities first. Yet again, energetic imbalances may be similarly amenable to acupuncture as a measure of first recourse. However, in any case of multifaceted or systemic issues that have as part of their overall picture a muscular component, redress of that muscular component by somatic education may be the "foot in the door" that interrupts the cycle and paves the way for a new trajectory toward healing and wellness.

While on the topic of medical conditions attributed to structural causes, it is not uncommon for clients to arrive for somatics services toting along with them some previously assigned medical label or diagnosis that purportedly identifies their problem. Certainly, on occasion, this can be helpful as we somatics practitioners need to know if a client suffers from a bone fide medical condition. Quite often, however, diagnostic labels prove to be inaccurate or misleading and even damaging to the extent that they create false expectations. Or else they merely label the presenting symptoms without casting helpful light on their underlying causes.

Inaccuracies can stem from outright misdiagnosis, diagnosis "by default" (...it's probably just a little arthritis), or they may be inadvertent, often resulting from a medical provider's need to fit a patient's diagnosis into an acceptable insurance category. Beyond the obvious problems stemming from incorrect diagnosis, labeling invites patients to identify with the known or presumed typical criteria of their diagnosis and to adjust their expectations for themselves accordingly. For example, if a client reports that he's been diagnosed with patellofemoral syndrome, or carpal tunnel syndrome, or any of a host of other musculoskeletal disorders, there may follow the assumption that the structural nature of diagnosis disqualifies the client as a suitable candidate for somatics.

The fact is that many conditions regarded as structural (and for which surgery might otherwise be indicated) resolve fully and easily with somatics. Clients, therefore, should be circumspect in how invested they allow themselves to become in any medical diagnosis, especially if the diagnostic label fails to enhance their prospects for recovery.

Other common conditions, aside from the aforementioned structural or neurological concerns, for which somatics is understood to have limited value may include, well, anything not having to do with muscles, either directly or indirectly.

Though I expound at length about the suitability of somatics for clients, both young and old, another important consideration is the suitability of any given individual client for somatics. Because somatic education entails a collaborative learning process between client and provider, clients who expect to have their needs met by the practitioner, but who are not prepared or equipped to share fully in that process, will likely find that their experience falls short of expectations. In order for somatics to be optimally effective, clients must be prepared to shoulder their full share of responsibility in participating, and in following up according to the advice of their practitioner. The same caveats apply for clients whose expectations surpass reason.

Though the techniques and methodologies defining the somatics approach are decidedly different from those ascribed to by massage, chiropractic, or other popular therapeutic modalities, the enduring efficacy of somatics can just as easily hinge on factors extrinsic to the client as with any other discipline. There are any number of possible *obstacles to cure*. Specifically, unhealthy lifestyle considerations can undermine, even sabotage, the somatics experience. For all its promise, somatics does fall somewhat short of magic. Lifestyle stressors—physical, emotional, or otherwise—that continue to exert their effects in a client's life can effectively prevent the client from gaining an appreciable or lasting benefit from somatics, or from any other therapeutic modality for that matter.

Imagine a more medically based scenario in which someone contracts asthma after moving into a dank, musty basement apartment. Whatever treatment that person seeks for relief is unlikely to produce lasting improvement if the client refuses to relocate into healthier quarters. At best, the symptoms may be suppressed by asthma medications. Or, imagine an individual with chronic back pain caused by daily heavy manual labor. Absenting a reprieve from the causative factor—heavy labor—even somatics will likely prove a Band-Aid at best. In his archived lectures, Thomas Hanna recounted how he had several rodeo cowboys as clients whom he maintained as shipshape for riding competitions as best he could, even though they regularly took bad spills during their rodeo events.[2] It's not difficult to imagine how such ongoing, albeit self-induced, physical abuse could countermand the gains engendered by the somatics approach.

It is also noteworthy that in his retelling of these clients' circumstance, Dr. Hanna highlighted the value of somatics not only as an agent of corrective measures, but also its potential for preventative care and ongoing maintenance. Even in such cases as described above, somatics can teach people how to use their bodies more intelligently to reduce the likelihood of new injury or the severity of relapse into old problems. I have worked with a number of

---

2 Thomas Hanna's archived lectures, June 29, 1990. CD #9.

tradespersons who have reported exactly that: as a result of their HSE experience they have learned how to use their bodies more intelligently while on the job to reduce the occurrence of previously recurrent problems. Somatics can effectively address a wide range of neuromuscular issues, but in the end it is the client's responsibility to insure that his or her lifestyle doesn't sabotage the positive effects of the somatics experience.

The only other limitation of note that comes to mind has to do with client compliance in keeping up the prescribed home practice movement patterns, and doing them in a correct manner. I repeat: somatics can work wonders for many people, but not beyond any extent to which clients are prepared to assume full responsibility for their person.

PART 2

APPLIED SOMATICS

To illustrate the broad efficacy of somatics I'd like to share the personal accounts of three individuals, each of whose lives has been touched deeply by somatics.

Account #1, Marilyn

As a child, Marilyn twisted her lower back and sacroiliac while trying to stand up from a backbend position. She lived with her pain for more than forty-five years. Her doctor originally diagnosed "growing pains" that would subside on their own. But the pains didn't subside. As an adult she navigated between medical doctors, chiropractors, and physical therapists for years with scant relief.

By the time Marilyn entered into her early fifties, her kids were on their own and she found herself bristling at the prospect of a lifetime of pain ahead such as she'd endured for the first half of her life. Serendipity knocked when her newly arrived copy of *Massage Therapy Journal* slipped from her grasp and fell open on the floor to an article about a "Radical Bodyworker." The accompanying photo that showed a kindly looking older man caught her attention.

It turned out the man in the article maintained a clinic within driving distance. Alas, a phone inquiry revealed he was booked up solid for a year in advance! But he did have room in an upcoming workshop that Marilyn was able to attend. As luck would have it, Marilyn's posture was so obviously poor that the workshop presenter, one Dr. Thomas Hanna, called upon her as a demonstration model. The few minutes she spent on Dr. Hanna's table were enough to change her life completely. Although there was some immediate improvement, it was her regular home practice of the simple movement patterns she'd learned on Hanna's table that provided the real turning point. While practicing at home one evening Marilyn experienced a breakthrough. "I felt as though someone's hands were on my hips, rotating the left hip backward and the right on forward, at which point my whole lumbar spine and pelvis cracked loudly and the pain was instantly gone!" Forty-five years of back pain subsided in a single crescendo.

Account #2, Steve

As young college student, Steve was diagnosed with both fibromyalgia and chronic fatigue syndrome. Here is his personal account.

It was in my early years in high school that I first starting experiencing symptoms, although I wasn't aware of them as symptoms as such at the time. I was just always tired and prone to achiness. When I started my first year of college I began to notice even more that I was sore and achy all the time; it was getting worse. My back was in constant pain and my body was extremely tender. Just sitting on the bench in my art class left me feeling bruised and incapacitated. Even playing the piano in music class hurt my wrists and forearms.

I sought out the medical opinions of my primary care physician and my chiropractor. I told my doctor it was clear was that something just wasn't right. Here I was still a teenager and already feeling old and frail. He responded that, "I wasn't old and I would be just fine." My condition continued to deteriorate.

During the summer after my first year at college I worked at a New Age bookstore where I found myself leafing through a book titled *Somatics*, which seemed to deal with the structure and design of the human body in a very sensible way. Given my own interest in industrial design, this idea of working with the body according to its design appealed to me. Unfortunately, my initial attempts to find a somatics practitioner proved futile.

During my second year of college I was diagnosed with both fibromyalgia and chronic fatigue syndrome, and by the spring of my third year I was basically disabled. I had to drop out of college and move back into my parents' house. It was that spring that I finally found, and first saw, a Hanna somatics practitioner. My first clinical session seemed inconclusive with no dramatic improvement, yet I somehow felt myself a little better for the experience. After so many years of chronic tightness in my legs they felt looser as I walked. Over the next several months I continued to see steady improvement from our sessions; and I also undertook to practice the somatics movement patterns depicted in the book *Somatics*, which contributed also to my improvement.

My symptoms gradually subsided over a three-year period until, eventually, I pronounced myself symptom-free. Looking back, I credit the combined effects of both clinical work with an excellent practitioner and my near-religious adherence to home practice exercises as being responsible for my gradual recovery over an extended period. Of all the different approaches I tried, Hanna somatics had the greatest impact in healing my musculoskeletal symptoms and relieving my chronic fatigue.

Account #3, Karen

Karen's passion was for math and physics. One day, at age twenty-four, while Karen was driving, a pedestrian stepped out in front of her car. Karen slammed on her brakes and veered for what seemed like an eternity, but was unable to avoid a collision.

Following this accident, Karen was out of work, briefly, due to the trauma to her own body. She began experiencing intermittent, but severe, pain in her right knee. Over the next ten years Karen sought advice from eight different physicians as she was shuffled through the medical system. Doctor after doctor recommended she succumb to knee surgery, ostensibly to clean up her damaged cartilage. Eventually Karen opted for knee surgery.

According to the post-surgical assessment report, the surgery was a success. Yet Karen was worse off than before. For the next year she required a cane or crutches to maneuver short distances around her house. Anything more called for a wheelchair. It wasn't long before her doctors were chomping at the bit to get back into her knee, but Karen was reticent. Instead, she sought relief in other less conventional therapies: energy therapy, acupuncture, Zero Balancing work, Traeger work, Shen Therapy, and Feldenkrais. None of these helped.

After about a year of this, one of the counselors at her women's health center suggested she consult with Thomas Hanna, a reputed whiz at musculoskeletal problems. Karen looked into this referral and learned that Hanna was a doctor of philosophy, of all things, not even a physician. Her first impression was that this was not a good sign, considering all the learned medical minds she'd consulted in the past. However, she read Hanna's book and was persuaded to follow up by his recounting of successes in working with patient after patient whose storyline roughly paralleled her own.

Dr. Hanna took one look at her and surmised that she'd undergone some sort of traumatic physical event about ten years prior (actually, eleven years). Hanna showed Karen how she had been living with the right side of her body profoundly compressed. For more than a decade her ribs had been pressed tightly down against her pelvis. He also showed her that the relative levels of her two shoulders were quite off. These were issues that been present in Karen's body since the original accidents but which none of her consulting physicians had picked up on.

Dr. Hanna began by establishing her "before" range of motion according to several planes. Then he proceeded with a standard protocol he'd developed for her type of condition. After Hanna completed a right-sided Lesson 2 (Trauma protocol), Karen experienced for the first time since her accident a full and healthy range of motion in her body. She was immediately pain-free. In fact, on leaving her session she walked unassisted down the stairs from Hanna's office. Once at the bottom of the stairs Karen turned around and walked all the way back up the stairs, and then excitedly scampered again down to the stoop. There she sat and burst into tears.

Karen went back for one more session with Dr. Hanna to clear up a separate issue (some tightness in her lower back that he forecast would haunt her in another ten years if left unattended). However, from that first session onward she remained pain-free and never relapsed.

Each of these three case accounts began or took place more than twenty years ago. And each of these three individuals was so enamored of their early experiences with Hanna somatics that they undertook professional training to pursue careers as somatic educators. These three individuals are Marilyn War-nock, Steve Aronstein, and Karen Hewitt, my trainers at the Somatic Systems Institute, and sources of guidance and inspiration that I will always cherish.

CHAPTER 7

SOMATICS AND SPORTS

We live in a culture that places a high value on sports and fitness. Of course, not everyone ascribes to an active sporting and fitness lifestyle. But those who do often display enough enthusiasm to more than make up for folks on the sidelines. Unfortunately, being active and being smart/healthy/active are not the same thing. Many of the activities currently popular with fitness enthusiasts are of questionable value when it comes to the "smart" and "healthy" parts of health and fitness.

The great majority of competitive sports and many noncompetitive fitness activities are notoriously hard on the body, regardless of whether they occur at the level of professional or amateur performance. The potentially most damaging of all on the body are those that are both high-impact, and high-contact (as in contact against others). Among the more popular of these are football, basketball, soccer, hockey, martial arts, and, of course, boxing and its ilk.[1]

Athletes who participate on a professional level place themselves under tremendous pressure to continually push their bodies to the limits of endurance and beyond. Weekend warriors seeking to emulate their professional idols can be even more susceptible to injury because their bodies are usually less well conditioned. Injuries resulting from high-impact, high-contact sports are common and can be serious. Quite often the momentum of play and the drive to perform take precedence over better judgment where health maintenance and recuperation from injury or fatigue may be concerned.[2] De-

---

1 The boxing "ilk" includes any sport in which part of the goal entails participants trying to injure, versus merely out-perform, one another.
2 Seth Mnookin, "When to Hang It Up," *Boston Globe Magazine*, 5/6/07.

spite the fact that most of the sports represented in this category have an off season, it is rare to see professional careers extend far beyond age thirty with high-impact and high-contact sports. More often than not, the rigors of the sport catch up with someone by then. Those Nolan Ryan, George Foreman, and Martina Navratilova types whose professional careers extend into their forties or beyond are certainly the exception rather than the rule.

A slightly less demanding category of sports are medium- to high-impact and non- or low-contact. Sports in this category include tennis, bowling, baseball, running, track and field, skiing, and some aspects of martial arts. At least three of these are, or can be, primarily unilateral, meaning they emphasize the use of one side of the body disproportionate to the other. Even with these activities, competitive careers usually wind down before age thirty-five. Though the potential for jarring physical contact so characteristic of the earlier category is less pronounced here, injuries are still common with these sports due to the frequency and extent to which players push their bodies beyond their limits.

Noncompetitive fitness activities that are medium- to high-impact comprise yet another level of activity demand. Here we include dance, martial arts,[3] weightlifting, recreational skiing, and working out at a gym, among others. That enthusiasts may not compete regularly against other individuals or teams hardly mitigates the drive to perform or succeed. The mindset with which one dances or lifts weights may still compel enthusiasts to explore beyond or exceed the limits of their bodies.

Finally, there is a low-impact category, including golf, yoga, biking,[4] swimming, and Taijiquan. Practiced recreationally, these activities are gen-

---

3 Martial arts, because of its many facets and different interpretations, can be experienced at different levels of physical demand. The more rigorous demands of combat training differ from those of individual practice or of choreographed techniques, and even more so from internal practices such as Tai Chi. Other sports, as well, can vary widely in the demands they place on the body.

4 Statistically, bicycling is one of the most dangerous sports, according to *LiveScience Health SciTech* online. Swimming and golfing also are rated in the top 15 for ER visits. In categorizing them thus, I am considering the effects of these sports on the body aside from concomitant dangers e.g., traffic, competition, etc.

erally less competitive and non-jarring. Some of them include an inherent mind/body component, which in my way of thinking not only shifts them out of the "not bad for you" category, but actually contributes to an overall sense of health and well-being, even above and beyond the cardiovascular and muscle-toning benefits commonly attributed to the other categories of activities mentioned.

Somatics is uniquely suited to meet the special needs of individuals whose bodies regularly endure the challenges and rigors of any and all sporting and fitness activities. Having arranged these many activities according to their respective categories, I assure you that somatics clinical work and regular practice of somatics movement patterns will, at the very least, contribute to enhanced performance and more rapid recovery for enthusiasts of every sport listed in every category mentioned above. How so?

First, you may wonder why I went through the motions of establishing these hierarchical categories at all if only to assert that their devotees share equally in candidacy as somatics clients. I opted for this tack because somatics, for all its efficacy in addressing current or preexisting neuromuscular problems or imbalances, can offer no guarantee against the occurrence of future injuries. No matter that some individual may engage in somatics to resolve an injury (or even practice somatic movement patterns on a daily basis for maintenance and prevention of injuries) to engage in risky behavior includes the likelihood of incurring injury. Somatics can reduce this likelihood and the possible severity of certain types of injuries incurred during times of physical rigor. But, if you engage in risky or demanding activities, your body can't avoid experiencing the consequences of those demands. The higher you go on the impact/contact scales noted above, the greater the likelihood that something will happen to you caused by forces beyond your immediate control. Such inherent risk is surely part of the allure of these sports for adrenaline junkies.

Despite this allure, sports offering the prospect of high impact and hard contact do constitute one possible obstacle (remember "obstacles to cure"?)

to the ongoing health and well-being of your body. Am I indicting them as such? No way, except for those "sports" in which part of the goal is to injure your opponent. I've already revealed myself as a martial arts professional. I also happen to be a tennis enthusiast. And I love to get out and hit the dance floor every now and then. I've been a rock climber and a scuba diver. I took up surfing in my fifties, and I occasionally sidle about on a Ripstick. I like to feel my body perform and to push the envelope a bit. Somatics helps my body continue to perform to the best of its ability even though I'm more than forty years into a career field known for its physical demands on the body. My position is that there is a cause-and-effect relationship to be considered with all physical activities, and anything you can do to turn the odds in your favor should prove a welcome addition to your overall training ethic. Though the hierarchical categories described represent an escalating level of risk to your body, somatics can, in many cases, help you to avoid injuries of a neuromuscular nature, and recover from them more quickly and fully if they do occur to avoid their long-term consequences.

When I think of the athletes whose careers have been severely impacted or cut short by neuromuscular pain and limitation—just in the tennis world, Pete Sampras, Andre Agassi, Kim Clisters, and Justine Henin come to mind—I feel deeply impassioned by the potential of somatics to manage or eliminate pain and improve performance.

In the case of professional athletes, for whom downtime due to injuries can mean more than mere inconvenience, somatics not only helps prevent injuries, but also offers the prospect of a much accelerated recovery. Professional athletes and sports teams that adopt somatics into their training programs will find its benefits to be more than cost-effective.

Every sport mentioned in the above hierarchy, plus some not listed, requires of its participants a certain level of performance. In the words of

Thomas Hanna, "A perfect athlete is a person who has full control...full voluntary cortical control of the striated muscles of the body."

"Performance" is just another way of saying you have that control and that your body cooperates and does your brain's bidding. Performance means that the muscles of your motor system do what your brain tells them to do, exactly. Obviously, your brain stands to gain more cooperation and response from muscles that are "smart" and able to do its bidding than it does from muscles that are proprioceptively illiterate. Enhanced proprioceptive literacy—meaning smarter muscles—is exactly what somatics is designed to help you achieve.

Of equal concern to every athlete should be the issue of normal and regular maintenance. Assuming your muscles have cooperated, and your day on the court, field, or dance floor, etc., is behind you, do you find yourself prone to soreness, aka "weekend warrior" syndrome? The usual response to aches and pains might be to take a hot soak, or seek out some deep tissue massage, or opt for analgesics; or you might simply wait out the interval until your soreness subsides.

Part of what contributes to this aftermath is any degree to which muscles that you've worked hard have, in turn, failed to stand down and really relax. Other than where there is normal lactic acid accumulation or simple fatigue, any place in your body where there is evidence of any degree of sensorimotor amnesia is exactly where one is most likely to experience discomfort, and where normal soreness from overwork is more often exacerbated. Localized SMA produces localized discomfort. More generalized sensorimotor amnesia will produce more generalized discomfort. Simple. Of course, mere exhaustion, muscle fatigue, or bruises, etc., can also be implicated.

Not every occurrence of pain indicates sensorimotor amnesia. But many pains are harbingers, serving as evidence of insults destined to culminate in SMA. This may beg the question of how one might recognize sensorimotor amnesia as distinct from acute, self-resolving, muscle pain or soreness. Generally, sensorimotor amnesia involves some element of muscular habituation and is best pinpointed by providers trained in recognizing its particular characteristics. That said, if there are lingering pains or discomforts, the likelihood is that the body has some degree or other of SMA. Chapter 11 addresses the subject of sensorimotor amnesia and muscular habituation in greater technical detail.

Generally, if you get in the habit of both preparing for and following up demanding activity sessions with some time dedicated to simple somatics movement patterns you will find that you will be less prone to soreness, and that much or all of whatever discomfort you do incur resolves more rapidly, including those issues not directly stemming from sensorimotor amnesia. Taking a few minutes for somatics practice prior to martial arts training or a tennis match makes a big difference for me, both in how my body performs and in how I feel and recover afterwards. In addition, somatics will help you enjoy the distinct advantage of knowing you are more in control of your body, and that you are better able, on your own, to implement simple measures that reduce pain and discomfort. You'll be more in charge of yourself. This can be a source of comfort for anyone, but particularly for older athletes who might otherwise be inclined to reduce activity levels as the anticipatory demands of exercise on their body come to feel increasingly inconvenient and limiting.

Finally, there is the issue of recovery from outright injuries. For athletes who love the feeling of exercising their bodies, few experiences are more disheartening than being out of commission. Many somatics movements can be integrated right into an overall recuperative strategy. This is significant in two regards. First, because the movement patterns of somatic education are slow and mindful, they are generally safe. It's almost impossible to overdo it when you practice somatics correctly. Why sit around and do nothing while your body heals on its own if you can just as easily contribute actively to a faster (complication-free) recuperation and make your muscles smarter in the process? Somatics movement patterns are benign and adjustable enough that they can be customized to many a healing process.

Second, the surgical interventions often necessitated by injuries are, themselves, detrimental to your body (think major insult here). Regardless of how necessary or indicated a surgical intervention may be, even in some circumstance of a lifesaving procedure, cutting open one's body still represents a significant insult. Any injury of note, as damaging as it may be by itself, is certain to be accompanied by concomitant (side effect) issues as the body attempts to compensate (recall Joe in Chapter 5) for limitations brought about by the injury. Sometimes these compensatory effects can linger long beyond the point that the original injury has resolved. Given these considerations, somatics (whether simple movement patterns or clinical sessions) can aid in both the speed and efficacy of almost any recovery process.

Individual and Unilateral Sports

Golf, bowling, and singles tennis are sports that come immediately to mind as placing disproportionate demands on either side of the body. I've only occasionally golfed or bowled, but I'm an avid tennis player when I'm not teaching Tai Chi or seeing clients in my clinic. These sports have in common a certain unilaterality in the demands they place on the body. As players' bodies respond to those demands, the unilateral nature of the activity can evidence itself in their bodies both on and off the playing area. Naturally, the extent to which this occurs can vary from individual to individual, depending on any number of factors: How long has someone been playing? Does that person play infrequently or often? Does he or she balance time on the playing court, lanes, or golf course with other non-unilateral activities that might tend to offset the imbalances caused by swinging a racquet, club, or heavy ball repeatedly from just one side of the body? What are the cumulative effects of other sources of stress on someone's body when factoring in work, family, etc.?

Bearing in mind that tennis, bowling, and golf each require an extraordinary level of control and precision to play well and successfully, the effects of even small imbalances in one's game can compromise performance beyond an acceptable level. Somatics can correct many preexisting neuromuscular imbalances caused by overuse of one side of the body to the exclusion of the other and effectively prevent the entrenchment in your body of new imbalances. Somatics can also help athletes improve their self-sensing abilities and bodily control. With these sports as examples of activities that require precise control, the advantages of developing more intelligent muscles should be self-evident.

For sports or fitness activities that are less physically rigorous and jarring, such as Tai Chi or yoga or recreational swimming, somatics can be every bit as helpful. Tai Chi and yoga, in particular, entail a mindful quality that makes somatics the perfect companion practice because somatics, like yoga and Tai Chi, encourages intrapersonal awareness through conscious self-sensing. It might seem an oversimplification to say as much; but many people undertake these activities because they aspire to be somehow different, to be better than they already are. They recognize a need or desire for change, often based on some perception of bodily limitation. Yoga enthusiasts or Tai Chi'ers can spend decades trying to evolve beyond the physical barriers imposed by their own preexisting sensorimotor amnesia (recall that SMA generally occurs at a level below conscious awareness) without ever realizing that SMA is the root cause of their limitations. Somatic education can be a godsend for yoga enthusiasts or Tai Chi'ers, especially for those who have hit a plateau in their practice. Even with a background in yoga or Tai Chi, the brain can only precisely control those muscles it can sense. Somatics is the perfect tool for the perfect job in shaving years or decades off the task of sensing and becoming able to really "know" and control your own body for an enhanced quality of life. Somatics is truly "meditation for your body."

My colleague, Karin Scholz Grace, M.S., took initiative in combining aspects of Hanna somatics with yoga, which she teaches and has practiced for more than twenty-five years. Following a traffic accident, in which she was hit by a truck while riding her bicycle, Karin suffered for years from chronic neck and back pain that yoga alone failed to resolve. Hanna somatics changed all that by providing her the means to release her muscular tension and restore her body to wellness. Karin has since developed her own brand of somatic yoga, which she describes as a safe, gentle style utilizing somatic principles of inward sensing and conscious rebalancing of the body. Her somatic yoga uses slow, mindful movement to prepare for poses (asanas), and explore skeletal alignment and muscle action within poses. Karin finds that yoga asanas become easier, safer, and more natural when agonist/antagonist groups are working in harmony, and unconscious holding is released.

"In somatic yoga," she says, "we begin working outside of the requirements of being upright against gravity, exploring activation and inhibition of muscles in safe positions that allow exploration without undue strain. Gradually we integrate the new muscular patterns into more challenging asanas, maintaining the neuromuscular balance alongside greater demands for strength, balance, and coordination."

She goes on to explain, "Yoga, as commonly practiced in this country, can overemphasize the yang qualities of effort and muscle action; the yin qualities of surrender and receptivity are forgotten in the yogi's commitment to master demanding poses and form a particular shape with the body. Traditional yoga, as articulated by Patanjali, shares many core principles with Hanna somatics, particularly its teachings on inward focus and self-sensing, and an emphasis on ease, comfort, and relaxation. Because these teachings are not brought to the fore in most yoga training in the West, Hanna somatics as an adjunct practice can focus the spotlight on this crucial aspect of the yogi's practice, giving us deeper mastery of the art of conscious relaxation. In a context where we are not attempting to form a particular shape, but instead are guided only by our internal sensation, we learn to promote muscle lengthening by voluntarily inhibiting muscle tension, rather than learning to use force to stretch a habitually contracted muscle. By creating balance between action and surrender, effort and ease, Hanna somatics reinforces the paradigms of harmony and attunement, which are fundamental to yoga practice.

"Hanna somatics is beneficial for experienced yogis, bringing deeper levels of awareness and mind-body performance to their practice; it can also bring the fundamentals of yoga to those who have never practiced the art. Those of us with limitations from injuries or illness may lack the strength, flexibility, or coordination required for even basic yoga asanas. Hanna somatics safely brings many of the benefits of yoga to people who may not be ready for yoga class. Somatic yoga, drawing on standard Hanna somatics movement principles and patterns, encourages students to develop into traditional yoga asanas, thoroughly preparing their bodies for the challenges, and instilling the powerful practice of respectful mindfulness."

I will comment in greater detail in Chapter 11 on the advantages of somatics for Tai Chi'ers and martial artists in general. Aside from its application to yoga and martial arts, HSE can enhance one's performance in a range of other sport and fitness disciplines.

As a brain/body educational resource, somatics is unique in its overall approach and efficacy as a sports and fitness adjunct, regardless of the sport or activity in question. Certainly, in the case of any given sport that entails contact or jarring, somatics can assist you in achieving peak performance by eliminating factors that cause hindrance, and by optimizing sensorimotor communication. Participation in other sports as well can only be improved by the prospect of enhanced proprioception and a reduced likelihood of injury. Athletes who incorporate somatics into their daily lives will be less susceptible to injuries; they will extend their playing careers and take more pleasure in their activities, knowing that minor problems can be managed or avoided altogether and that major problems are less likely to mean an end to staying active.

To illustrate these points further I have included several case histories that deal with sports-related issues drawn from the files of somatic education professionals.

Case #1. Footballer with a Back and Pelvis Injury

This case was solicited via interview with Jonathan Hunt, a Hanna somatics colleague with a clinical practice in England. Jonathan's situation echoes my own in that he suffered an injury that eventually led him to pursue somatics as a career choice.

During the 1990s, Jonathan was a top pro footballer in England. His professional career, which included Premiership status, spanned some twelve years. He played for Wimbledon and other clubs until his career was cut short at age twenty-nine by an injury suffered during football play.

Jonathan's account is simple, yet poignant. While he was playing football (aka soccer) he made a challenge for the ball during routine play. Rather suddenly he experienced a sharp sensation of pain in his pelvic region. As Jonathan described it, the pain was immediately localized and excruciating. At the time his team's medical personnel gave him what treatment they could, but to no avail. Jonathan was referred to the hospital, where x-rays and a scan confirmed that he had shorn off the right adductors attached to his pelvis, with consequent inflammation of the pubic symphysis.

Over the next several months Jonathan's symptoms subsided somewhat, but only marginally. His pelvic injury seemed to resolve, but the pain worsened as it gravitated up into his lower back. The doctors at the hospital determined that he had prolapsed discs between L3-L4 and L4-L5, and surmised that, his recent trauma notwithstanding, the degenerative condition of his spine was more likely a long-term result of Jonathan's football career. In other words, the recent injury was just incidental to a more comprehensive under-lying issue. The hospital advised a surgical procedure for his lower back but Jonathan deferred, preferring to explore for non-surgical healing alternatives.

Over the next two years Jonathan's condition failed to improve substan-tively. He was considerably worse off in any circumstance that required sitting or, especially, driving, though moving about afforded some small measure of relief. Jonathan's condition was complicated by insomnia as his pain during this period made sleep nearly impossible. Among the various therapeutic mo-dalities Jonathan experimented were; shiatsu massage, acupuncture, manipu-lative physiotherapy, osteopathy, massage, cranial-sacral, and pilates. Most of-fered some temporary relief, only to have the pain recur shortly with renewed intensity. The pilates that was recommended by his doctor to strengthen his core, in particular only served to create a feeling of rigidity with a vice-like grip across Jonathan's center, ultimately aggravating his condition.

Some two years after his initial injury Jonathan took a holiday trip to Thailand. The day before his scheduled departure a friend advised him to visit an émigré, Cynthia Lindway H.S.E., who maintained a local practice in Hanna somatics. Due to his imminent departure she worked with him more intensively, consolidating aspects of several somatics protocols into a single long session. The measure of relief Jonathan experienced from that first initial session was substantial, immediately producing more improvement in his condition than all his previous treatments combined. By his own account, Jonathan estimated a seventy percent reduction in pain and discomfort from that one session. He was sufficiently inspired by this experience that he opted for a return trip to Thailand six weeks later for additional work. This, and his follow-up with regular practice at home on his own, satisfactorily resolved Jonathan's outstanding pain issues.

Jonathan's success with somatics prompted him to pursue professional training at the Novato Institute to become a certified Hanna somatic edu-cator. Currently, Jonathan maintains a Hanna somatics practice for people, and an adjunct practice in equine somatics. He remains free of the constant pain that characterized his life for two years following his injury. He is quite confident that the thirty–sixty minutes he spends each day practicing somatics movement patterns on his own will suffice in keeping him free of relapse.

After five years out of the game, Jonathan resumed playing football, albeit at a semiprofessional level, two or three times weekly. Additionally, Jonathan is active with golf and long-distance running, and is considering triathlons. He asserts that his fitness levels are as high, if not higher, than before because somatics afforded him a greater freedom of movement, quicker recovery times, and greatly enhanced breathing, all issues he recalls having struggled with during his earlier professional football days. "Somatics," Jonathan affirms, "would have greatly enhanced my professional playing career both physically and emotionally."

Case #2. Young Female with a Running Injury

The following case was submitted by my HSE colleague, Martha Peterson (Bixler). Martha maintains a private practice in New Jersey. [Note: Client name is fictional to protect client privacy.]

Sandra was a star runner for a collegiate track team, having earned All-American honors in cross-country running. In her last major race at the National Championships she ran an under-eighteen-minute 5,000 meter. Then she suffered a serious overuse injury to her psoas muscle. Fearing she would never run again, Sandra consulted a number of different practitioners: physical therapists, doctors, orthopedists, and massage therapists, to no avail. All parties were in agreement that her psoas was tight and clearly implicated in her pain, but no one knew what to do about it. Sandra heard about somatics through a local health and wellness networking group. By the time I saw her she'd been sidelined from serious competition for almost a year.

Sandra and I worked together fairly consistently over the course of six weeks. Her complaints were very specific and right-sided: pain in the right hip/groin, hip flexors and right buttock down the right leg. A visual assessment showed that her left foot was slightly inverted, and she held her right arm slightly out from her body. She had an exaggerated sway in her back, and tended to lock her knees. Her left latissimus were pulled back as well, creating a twist in her torso.

She'd had an appendectomy (almost ruptured) and at one point broke both arms. She'd been running indoor track competitively, always training and running to the left. Her repetitive left-sided training seemed to explain what I saw in her left lats/shoulder area.

We started with Lesson 3 to address the psoas issue. I added some right-side trauma work as well. She reported that the next day she was sore, but following that she reported no pain at all! We proceeded with Lesson 1, right side, to address the exaggerated sway in her back. Her left shoulder was pulled back and down, pushing her right hip forward. During the next session we worked with her waist muscles (Lesson 2) on the left side, and I guided her through some somatic exercises (Lesson 8–walking lessons, from *The Myth of Aging* series) briefly to see what was going on with her pelvis. She'd had a lot of SMA in her lower lats, so I knew we would have to return to that side for more work.

We repeated Lesson 2, left side, and she really seemed to get some big releases! We added some pelvic basket rocking so that she could become more aware of the way her pelvis should be able to move. I guided her through some hip and shoulder rotations and more walking exercises. Subsequently, she reported back to me that she'd gone to a clinic where they filmed her running cadence and remarked that her stride and form were perfect! I advised her to get back to running slowly, first focusing with awareness on how she walked, before proceeding into a slow run. We finished up her sessions with a Lesson 1 on the left side. Sandra reported back that she was feeling terrific with no more pain when running. She said she does her daily home practice exercises faithfully.

The next running season Sandra was back on the track team. She wound up becoming the top seeded runner and captain of her team, and commented to me that were it not for Hanna somatics she would never have made a comeback at all. Two years after our first session, Sandra reported still feeling great. The sway in her back was practically gone and her posture remained comfortable and balanced.

Case #3. Recovery from Knee Surgery

The following is my own first-person account of surgical recuperation.

In the early stages of writing this book I had arthroscopic knee surgery, having incurred a tear to my left medial meniscus some eight months prior. The damage was idiopathic, though likely abetted by competitive tennis. In the months leading up to surgery my knee felt occasionally compromised in its lateral stability. My most prominent and limiting symptom was that full flexion of the knee (e.g., when I stooped low to sit back on my heels) was painful. I felt a total loss of that leg's weight-bearing ability while the knee was fully flexed, such as when I sought to balance myself on one foot while in a crouched sitting position. Granted, this is not your run-of-the-mill type of demand, but it was problematic for me in the context of my martial arts.

Both before and immediately following surgery I followed my own recuperative protocol, eschewing prescription drugs and painkillers altogether, as well as any conventional physical therapy. Instead, I relied on homeopathic arnica and certain herbs. Those remedies notwithstanding, I was still recovering from a surgical procedure and a requisite amount of swelling and stiffness was inevitable. Over the next several days my knee proved quite manageable, as the swelling and stiffness reduced according to my body's own wisdom on its own timetable, slowly but steadily. The most challenging part of my recovery process proved not to be my knee, but the manner in which the rest of my body compensated for my knee's limitations during the recovery period. Admittedly, if I'd stayed off my feet completely and followed a less active lifestyle, my body may have had a good deal less to compensate for. But that's just not my style. Besides, that approach may have produced its own set of problems, e.g., muscular atrophy. As a result, I felt discomfort, at times bordering on cramping, in my left calf and both thighs (albeit with different kinds of stresses in each thigh) as well as asymmetrical stresses in the muscles of my lower and middle back. My left thigh, in particular, felt very contracted due to the swelling, thus limiting my ability to flex the knee. My personal practice of somatics movement patterns proved invaluable in addressing these issues.

Starting on my second day post-op, I fashioned a series of self-pandiculations specific to the muscle functions involved. Using a belt under my toes to extend the reach of my arms, I practiced pandiculating my ankle from plantar-flexion into dorsa-flexion. Using a more rigid device, I practiced maneuvering my foot into plantar-flexion from a dorsa-flexed starting position. I practiced these articulations initially from a straight-legged position, in each case varying my plane of motion, first with the foot straight to the front, then internally rotated, then externally rotated. I also pandiculated my foot and ankle according to its ability to invert and evert. I repeated the same series of movements as I drew my foot incrementally closer while bringing my knee and hip into flexion. Several of the more standard somatics movement patterns were sufficient to address the discomforts stemming from tightness elsewhere in my body.

These various leg pandiculations, customized for my purposes, were instrumental in restoring range of motion to my ankle, knee, and hip. Within a week of surgery my knee was fully functional for all its usual and customary demands, and by ten days post-op I was back on the tennis court. I'd recovered about ninety percent of my range of motion, being able to flex my knee nearly to a point that I could touch heel to buttock. Plus, my knee felt quite stable in all directions. Certainly, my doctor and his medical team deserved a lot of credit. They did a superb job with my medical procedure. However, somatics played a major role in effectively restoring my body to peak performance condition and inhibiting what would surely have been my body's tendency, post-surgically, to add a compensatory layer of insult to my own personal archeology.

Summary

In reviewing the world of sports, skilled athletes often perform at or near peak performance even with bodies that may already be severely compromised, this in compelling testimony to their human potential, until some injury or condition sidelines them and prompts their seeking relief through corrective measures. I expect it is more the rule than the exception that most athletes, even though they may not be suffering from some full-blown limitation, are in some manner or other encumbered, causing their performance to be less than optimal.

Athletes are as subject as anyone else to the "archeology of insults" outlined in Chapter 1; so it's not a matter of *if* someone's body might be compromised, but merely a question of when and how badly. If skilled athletes are capable of outstanding performance with bodies that are compromised, just imagine how much better they might perform, or extend their playing careers by avoiding injury. If they could learn how to bring their bodies to a higher level of baseline health they'll be better able to muster on-demand peak performance. Somatics offers just that possibility and could be every athlete's best friend.

CHAPTER 8

THINK OF SOMATICS FOR...

I've emphasized throughout this text that somatics is not a medical modality. Somatics practitioners are not therapists; we are educators. This is a distinction we do not take lightly. As educators, our responsibility is not to keep you forever in the classroom, so to speak, but to coach you along to a point that you can graduate, to develop enough autonomy as regards your self-sensing abilities that you can become your own teacher. Our role is to teach individuals how to develop and maintain optimal communication between brain and body so that they may, ultimately, assume fuller voluntary control of their own body, even into old age. Granted, it is more than mere happy coincidence that the usual consequence of experiencing somatic education is to improve one's health and wellness overall. It is no fault of ours that people achieving health and wellness through our particular form of education may serve to highlight the differences between conventional therapeutic medicine and our alternative approach of providing people the means by which they can heal and maintain their own bodies. Perhaps conventional medicine, along with its sanctioned therapies, is not the only means by which people can effectively manage their health and well-being. Beyond teaching clients specific skills to improve themselves in ameliorating existing problems, our interest as somatic educators is in teaching clients how they themselves can learn to assume initiative whenever possible—in essence to become self-healers.

By asserting as much, it is not my intention to impugn or otherwise malign conventional medicine or therapeutic modalities. Many of the medical doctors I know, quite a number of whom are or have been students in my martial arts programs or clients in my Pain and Mobility Clinic, are open to and even excited about the prospects of non-conventional modalities in general, and somatics in particular. An encouraging trend amongst medical professionals is to recognize that conventional allopathic medicine does not have all the answers, or even the best answers for every circumstance, and that non-conventional approaches, such as somatic education, have much to offer.

It is certainly not a goal of somatics, as a powerful and emerging wellness resource, to alienate other healing modalities that hold a place at the table. I do not intend for any mean spirit or one-upmanship to stem from this camp. We merely raise our hands high and say, "Hey, everybody, we've got an approach, one with a practical and theoretical foundation in conventional neurophysiology that really works...stuff that nobody else seems to be doing! You ought to give this a try and see if it works for you."

All healing modalities have a time and a place according to the needs of the client, or patient. We providers, regardless of our chosen approach, should never lose sight of the fact that it is those needs, the needs of the client, that are paramount, regardless of the modality in question, and that all healing systems exist to serve the needs of the people, not vice versa. Sometimes healing systems, like governments, can lose sight of this simple fact—that they exist to serve their constituency. Ever mindful of this, somatic educators are here to help out as best we can. Somatics works quite well on its own—when that is just what the client needs. And somatics can also interface nicely as one part of a multi-modal approach—when that is just what the client needs. Providing effective healing services to others is all about determining the needs of the client, or patient, and then seeing to it that those needs are met. Our olive branch is thus extended to all who would effectively serve the health and wellness needs of our fellow man.

Since its introduction by Dr. Hanna, many people have found in somatics a powerfully effective resource in resolving a range of health and wellness issues. Usually, such resolve is direct, as when someone seeks out somatics to redress a particular issue. Other times the improvements that follow from somatics can be inadvertent. Early on in my clinical practice I had occasion to work with two different clients, each of whom stipulated complaints revolving around generalized muscular stress and tension but, primarily, it was back pain that brought them into my clinic. In addition to significant improvements with their back pain, each of these clients subsequently reported full or partial amelioration of concomitant conditions (surprise!). One fellow experienced substantial relief from his longstanding colitis, and the other from his Crohn's disease. In both cases their relief followed quickly on the heels of, and apparently in direct consequence to, their somatics work. The gentleman with Crohn's disease had failed to even mention this condition on his intake form or during our initial interview, so inured was he to its presence in his life. I only learned about it when, after his first two sessions, he mentioned excitedly, "By the way, my Crohn's disease has completely gone away since I started somatics." He never imagined any connection between his body's alimentary function and his more immediate neuromuscular complaints. Several months later the other gentleman informed me that in addition to his colitis having abated his restless leg syndrome, which had plagued him for some years, had subsided nearly completely, again seemingly as a result of practicing the somatics home practice patterns I taught him.

In contrast to the longstanding reductionist/mechanistic overview ascribed to by many of those who have been at the forefront of Western science and medicine since the time of Descartes, I feel it is important to operate from a premise that everything is connected. Certainly, even distal issues in the human body, more often than not, have roots tracing back to the core. This is one reason that we somatic practitioners generally eschew "spot work," or attending to just a symptomatic area to the exclusion of the whole. As a rule, we ascribe to a more integrated approach, working from the core of the body outward.[1]

Given the rationale that everything is connected, certain causations can be expected to result in certain predictable effects. Where my aforementioned

---

1   On rare occasions, a client's circumstance may dictate departure from this guiding principle, e.g., with my stroke client described in Chapter 6.

client might never have considered his muscular tension and stress to be a contributing factor, let alone a possible cause of his Crohn's disease, in somatics a nonlinear correlation such as this is entirely plausible. To reiterate, Green Light conditions are often characterized by a logical assemblage of symptoms, all of which are congruent with the stresses inherent to a Green Light posture. Red Light and Trauma postures are similarly predisposed to a predictable smorgasbord of symptoms in expression of their underlying causes.

This wisdom is borne out in the collective experience of a multitude of somatic educators as evidenced by the following accounts drawn from their clinical case files. These accounts illustrate the wide-ranging efficacy of somatics in directly addressing the problems of sensorimotor amnesia, and indirectly addressing health and wellness problems that may be caused or abetted by sensorimotor amnesia.

Case Histories

[Note: Client names are fictional to protect client privacy.]

Case #1. Acute Traumatic Event—Automobile Accident

(From the author's files)

Here is the fully resolved case of a client, Zack, male, age thirty, who had been in an automobile accident. While out driving with his youngster buckled safely into the seat beside him, Zack was hit from the driver's side and just to the back (T-boned) by another vehicle. The impact was hard enough that his vehicle was declared a total loss. Airbags did not deploy. Fortunately, Zack and his son escaped broken bones, internal injuries, and even lacerations; but afterward Zack complained of pain along with tightness and pressure in his upper and lower back, and of headaches.

Imagine how your own body might react if you saw, out of the corner of your eye, another car heading straight at you from the side. Your body would instinctively recoil and twist away to shield itself from the force of impact. In Zack's case he was additionally motivated to shield his child. On his arrival at my office, Zack presented with a posture fully commensurate with just such a response, indicating a clear case of Trauma reflex pattern.

Scanning, from the bottom up, I observed that Zack's right foot was drawn back an inch or so from being even with his left foot. This was the most distal expression of his Trauma posture [Figure 8-1]. The right side of his body, extending from foot to shoulder, was "torqued back," having contracted to recoil his left side away from the perceived danger. This also involved a discrepancy in Zack's arms alongside his body. His right arm and shoulder were lower and retracted compared to the left.

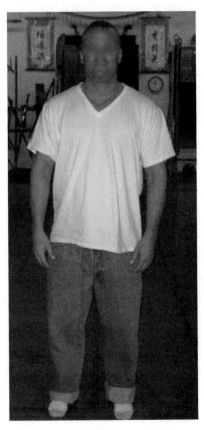

Figure 8-1.

Palpation confirmed a tightness running the length of Zack's right side. I opted to start him with a right-sided Lesson 2 Trauma session, which produced noticeable improvement. As his session unfolded, so did Zack. The muscles of his back became softer and more pliable and he commented on feeling his back and legs in a renewed way, "as if they were longer."

The torquing commensurate with his trauma posture was much ameliorated. However, as is sometimes the case, this improvement served to highlight the appearance of other, as yet unaddressed, imbalances. After his first session Zack's right shoulder was no longer depressed. In fact, that shoulder now appeared higher than the left shoulder. This was due to his newly apparent need for a Lesson 1 Green Light session. Not a matter of any great concern, this tilting was something I anticipated we would attend to during his next scheduled appointment. Following his first session, Zack reported immediate and substantial relief from his previous discomfort. I gave Zack a series of somatic movement patterns to practice at home over the next week to reinforce his gains.

On arrival for his second session, Zack reported new pains. Although the acute discomforts stemming from his accident were substantially diminished and his body was feeling much freer in its movement, he was now aware of pain in his right lower back and a feeling of constriction in his right shoulder. Questioning revealed that these pains were reminiscent of previous problems that predated his recent accident by some years, but that, apparently, had been held in abeyance by his weightlifting, which he had discontinued since his accident. He was only now experiencing a renewed awareness of these discomforts in follow-up to our previous session.

I explained to Zack that his somatics session hadn't "caused" these problems to reoccur; rather it merely revealed their latent presence. In all likelihood, the muscle tonus resulting from his years of weightlifting had functioned like a body splint (which also explained his inflexibility) to protect his body from its own painful condition. Due to our having unbound his body from this splinting layer of tight muscles during our initial session, his newly disencumbered body was now able to more fully experience some of the unresolved, albeit painful, issues we hadn't yet addressed—problems that had been in his body all along but which were only now reawakened from their dormancy. In all probability, these underlying issues would have remained dormant as long as they remained firmly splinted, for example until such time as Zack no longer lifted weights, at which time they would likely have reappeared with a vengeance. Had he not been introduced to somatics, Zack's life would probably have been a tradeoff between inflexibility and pain. Even barring his recent accident, Zack would have found himself eventually living with both inflexibility and pain. My goal was to help him escape both of these fates.

For our second session I opted for a Lesson 1, but on his right side due to the manner in which his body had acclimated to our earlier session. As part of this lesson I taught Zack additional exercise patterns for home practice. At the conclusion of our session, he reported feeling significant improvement in his shoulder and lower back.

After his second session Zack displayed marked improvement in his posture, overall [Figure 8-2]. His body was properly aligned vertically; his shoulders were level; his head sat straighter on his shoulders, and there was only a slight external rotation to the right foot. At this point I anticipated one additional session might be sufficient to resolve Zack's remaining issues.

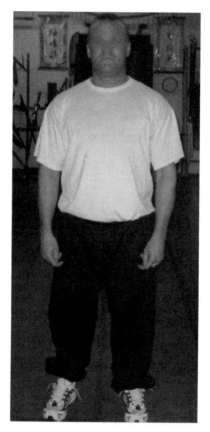

Figure 8-2.

As it turned out, Zack relapsed a bit before his final session due to his having felt sufficiently recovered to resume some ill-advised weightlifting. Even so, a final left-sided Lesson 2 effectively resolved his case. After Zack's third session his feet were symmetrical and nearly parallel. He displayed a vertical centerline, his body was free of torsion, and his head and neck sat straight atop his now nearly level shoulders [Figure 8-3].

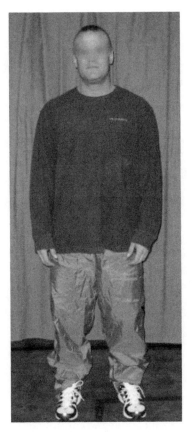

Figure 8-3.

From here on, it is Zack's responsibility to comply with home practice patterns to continually reinforce the gains he made. It should come as no surprise that Zack also reported, after his final session, utter amazement at the total absence of pain and discomfort in his back and shoulder.

Case #2. Effects of Whiplash Stemming from Auto Accident

(From the author's files)

Tina, forty-nine, is a close personal friend, and well familiar with the somatics I practice. Therefore, I was the first person she called after being rear-ended at forty mph by a teenager texting on her cell phone. The impact totaled Tina's Mercedes sedan.

I advised Tina to immediately contact her physician. She was already in considerable pain and her doctor advised her that the pain was likely to get worse over the next several days. Her doctor strongly urged her to forego any type of therapy for the time being. Despite her doctor's advice, Tina requested a somatics session ASAP.

She was extremely tender on arrival. The pain was localized to her neck muscles (scalenes and sternocleidomastoids). I began with a Green Light session, but Tina was in too much pain to tolerate the indicated maneuvers in a prone position. I opted instead to sit her upright in the same position she was in during the crash. From there I coaxed her through ten or fifteen minutes of very gentle, very simple assisted pandiculations for neck and shoulders. I didn't want to overdo it, given her tenderness.

On standing and moving about she felt much improved. I scheduled her for a follow-up session the next day, but she called in the morning to cancel as she felt only a mild residual soreness. Over the next several days I waited for another call, expecting some sort of relapse. It was two weeks later before she called, needing just a brief bit of follow-up work.

I wish this made for a more comprehensive and clinically impressive report, something with a bit of panache, but the truth is Tina's whiplash, serious by all accounts, was mostly resolved from a single abbreviated somatics session. That's the way it often goes with somatics.

Case #3. A Case of Frozen Shoulder

This case was submitted by my HSE colleague Jon Aronstein, a staff clinician at the Somatic Systems Institute.

My client, Beth, was a fifty-year-old female. She was experiencing a frozen left shoulder and suffered from general long-term low back and neck pain. She reported having injured her right (opposite) shoulder five years prior, to which she attributed her ongoing neck pain. Aside from her left shoulder, she seemed able to move freely without severe postural distortions. Mainly, she evidenced an internal rotation of her shoulders and a minor lordosis, with palpable tension in her low back and pectoral areas. Her left deltoid was rock hard, especially at the insertion area. She had extremely tight biceps on the left and her forearm was rotated medially. She tended to hold her elbow flexed at almost ninety degrees, and her scalenes and sternocleidomastoids were quite tight. Abduction of her arm away from her torso was limited to about twenty degrees. Any attempt to extend beyond that range produced excruciating pain in and below the deltoid area.

We began to address Beth's issues with a left-sided Trauma session. Initially, I spent quite a bit of time making tiny shoulder movements (means whereby) to acclimate her in preparation for larger motions and the full content of a Lesson 2 Trauma session. This first session seemed "plodding" and seemed to produce little improvement. Frankly, I was concerned by the degree of rigidity in the muscles around the shoulder. The shoulder and the elbow seemed almost structurally "fused." After this first session ended I reflected on Beth's situation and the approach I had taken, along with its (non)effects, and resolved to a different approach for our next scheduled session.

I was a bit nervous about her next session, but I kept that in check and opted to address her issues more from the center of her body than from the periphery. Session two entailed a Lesson 3, Red Light protocol. As it turned out, this suited her well. Beth was amazed at just how much range of motion we were able to accomplish by working around her pain rather than diving headlong into it. What seemed at the conclusion of her earlier session like a structural impediment was now clearly nothing more than tightness stemming from sensorimotor amnesia. By the end of her second session her arm movements were still jerky, but she was moving her arm. Just as importantly, Beth seemed to grasp the principles of slow, conscious movement as an important component for her own home practice. After two more sessions—a left-sided Lesson 1, Green Light session, and a repeat of her Lesson 2 on the left—Beth was able to abduct her arm all the way to ninety degrees, with minimal medial rotation while the arm hung at rest. At the end, she was quite pleased, as was I, with the outcome of her somatics sessions.

Case #4. Redressing Complications from Surgery, and More

This case was submitted by my HSE colleague, Laura Gates. Laura maintains a private practice in New York City.

The following case study focuses on the value of HSE as a recuperative resource for elderly clients recovering from surgery. Dave was eighty-five years old. He had undergone vascular surgery to his groin area on both sides to remove a blockage and repair a herniation in his aorta at the lower branch. For at least a year prior to surgery he suffered from considerable lack of circulation in his right leg. Symptoms included daily muscle spasms in the right calf, hip, and low back. Also, his leg gave way under him from time to time. According to his neurologist, this leg issue may have been due to a minor TIA (tiny broken blood vessel) in the back of the brain.[2]

Surgery provided some measure of improved circulation to Dave's leg, but the trauma of the surgery left his body bent forward a full forty-five degrees! Not surprisingly, this complication also resulted in low energy and shortness of breath. When Dave arrived for his first session, I noted that his

---

2 Transient ischemic attack, aka TIA.

left shoulder was pulled down, that he reported chronic pain and spasm in his right lower back. The heels of his shoes were worn badly on the outside due to his outwardly rotated feet, more so the right. He was still experiencing occasional calf spasms, and occasional loss of control of the right leg with collapsing, even though the circulation to that leg was reportedly somewhat improved. It seemed that the lack of circulation starved the muscles and nerves and that healing was progressing slowly as a result.

In the months following his surgery, we worked with the muscles of his legs and hips so that he might gain more cortical control and coordination of walking, increase blood flow, and speed up the healing process. In regards to his habituated forward bending, we pandiculated the psoas, and other hip flexors, abdominals, pectorals, and the front of his neck. Somatic movement pattern sequences included the Arch and Flatten, Arch and Curl, and the Diagonal arch/curl of shoulders to hip. After our first two sessions, Dave's flexion was improved from a chronic forty-five degrees to about five degrees. Also, the chronic pain in his right lower back resolved with pandiculation of the involved muscles, this by crossing the right leg over the left and letting both legs sink over to the left in stages. He continues to rely on that pattern when he feels any hint of the spasm returning. For the collapsed left side of his body, we pandiculated Dave's obliques and latissimus dorsi, as well as his upper and lower trapezius, and rhomboids. The somatic movement sequences, which I taught Dave to practice from a prone position, included a "diagonal waving motion of arms and legs," and the "diagonal lifting of arms, legs, and head." He reported these were especially helpful.

I suggested that Dave use a standing version of calf pandiculation whenever his calf bothered him while walking. He balanced against a mailbox or the like for support, while positioned in a lunge posture, his cramped leg straight and to the back. While in this position, he could lift his back heel to contract the gastrocnemius muscle and slowly release the contraction. I asked him to repeat the pandiculation with his back knee slightly bent to address any tightness in the soleus muscle as well. He could then reach down and use his hand to resist the foot that is flexing for reciprocal inhibition. I made flash cards with short somatic sequences to use in his chair or while reclining during the day and advised him to never stay seated for more than a half hour at a time without moving, as crossing of the legs and immobility both are clearly implicated in aggravating his problems. In addition, as his sleeping habit is to curl on the left side in a fetal position, I asked Dave to spend some of his sleeping time on his back, if possible, with supporting pillows under his knees.

Overall, somatics was most helpful in speeding Dave's recovery from this surgery. He no longer used a cane and his walking stamina slowly increased. In sum, he was very pleased with his change in posture and with the new tools he was given for curing his own lower back pain.

Case #5. The Story of Art's Mysterious Symptoms

The following case was submitted by my HSE colleague Lawrence Gold. Lawrence divides his clinical practice between Hawaii and Santa Fe, New Mexico.

Art came to me with an unusual story and an unusual set of symptoms illustrating that it isn't so much the injury, but the reaction to the sensations and perceptions that accompany an injury or threat that creates lasting problems.

A victim of a friend's foolishness in an automobile, Art arrived at my clinic displaying various neuromuscular symptoms and postural distortions typical of persons having suffered shock and injury. The shock and injury, in this case, occurred while Art was a passenger in his friend's car, which was moving at about fifty miles per hour. He was looking out the passenger side window while his friend was telling him how good the brakes were on his car. Without warning, his friend slammed on the brakes. Art had his seat belt on so, although he was pitched forward, he was restrained; even so, he reflexively braced himself with his right foot.

He came away from that incident with a complicated array of fixated muscular contractions, more on his right side than his left, dizziness, headaches, restricted breathing, numbness and weakness in the extremities, and tendencies of certain muscle groups to twitch or go into involuntary tightening in reaction to relatively mild changes of position. Following the incident, he often made shaking or kicking movements with his legs and shaking or thrusting movements with his arms to interrupt the twitching, which he found uncomfortable and disturbing, both emotionally and to his sleep.

The affected muscle groups included those of his neck, chest, back, and legs, with twists in his legs and pelvis—patterns that could reasonably be attributed to a whiplash injury that occurred with the head slightly turned and with a bracing action of the legs, which is what had happened.

Let's look at the array of symptoms and see how they correspond to the involved muscle groups: Dizziness and headaches are typical of restriction of the neck by muscular contractions. Headaches are caused both by physical pulls of tight neck muscles on the scalp and by reflexive responses. The dizziness in particular is interesting because conventional medicine has a hard time explaining the causative mechanism or dealing with it effectively. But if we understand dizziness as a result of malfunction of the brain-level reflexes that coordinate head movements (neck muscles), eye movements, and the balance centers of the inner ears, it makes perfect sense. We are designed to be able to visually follow objects while we and they are moving by using the coordination reflexes that link head movement to eye movement. These coordination reflexes are guided by the sensations of head movement produced by the balance centers of the inner ear. When neck muscles go into contraction, they provide an excessive sensation of movement to the brain, which leads to excessive movements of the eyes; they also distort head movements, which create unusual sensations of movement through the same balance centers. The result: dizziness, even when a person isn't in motion, known as "cervicogenic dizziness." This kind of neuromuscular reaction is known as Trauma reflex, a somatic response to pain or threat of injury.

Restricted breathing occurs when the muscles of breathing, particularly those between the ribs, go into contraction, as they might when we fall forward with crushing force against a seat belt in a sudden stop. This reflexive reaction, in which no discernible injury may have occurred but a painful sensation has occurred with suddenness, is a form of Trauma reflex.

Numbness and weakness in the extremities is a common result of nerve impingements (pinching), also resulting from muscular reactions in the neck and low back, arising from a shock reaction. In this case, another type of shock reaction, known as "startle" reflex (which takes a different form in adults than in infants) seems to have been involved. Startle reflex involves the act of contracting oneself in from the extremities, as if the body were curling into a ball or fetal position, resulting in predictable pathological muscular reflex patterns.

I interpreted Art's twitching since the incident as an automatic, sub-cortical adaptive response, which we can identify as the expression of a heightened state of readiness to react, as if always on the ready (i.e., a kind of hyper-reactivity, or hair trigger) for the next shocking situation to happen.

However, as understandable as these conditions might be to a clinical somatic educator, to correct them required more than skillful applications of clinical technique; it required some "detective work." Merely to have dealt with the muscular responses in terms of tight muscles or altered posture may have freed our client from the bulk of his postural distortions, but his reaction pattern involved more than the tightening of muscles; it was the tightening of muscles in a pattern. As it was, Art's condition came from both his reaction when his friend slammed on the brakes and the postural position he was in when it happened. So I asked Art to recall his position at the time of the incident. Sensorimotor amnesia often hides this information (just as, in many people, it veils any memory of having even had an injury). Once Art and I were able to reconstruct his position, we were able to apply the indicated somatic learning techniques to bring him relief from the twitching.

Art received significant relief during the few sessions we did. Even so, it was necessary for him to practice somatics exercises on his own to internalize and integrate the changes brought about during our clinical sessions.

Even in the absence of tissue damage, the shock of the stressing incident was sufficient to trigger in Art a host of somatic reactions, reactions similar to those often caused by genuine traumatic injury.

Case #6. A Case of Scoliosis

The following first-person account was submitted by my HSE colleague, Katherine Kerber.

I was born with scoliosis and a left leg that was "shorter" than my right leg. Luckily, my scoliosis formed an "S" curve, which meant that my spine was somewhat compensated. As a youngster, I was prescribed a lift in my left shoe to even out my hips. Throughout my teen years, I maintained an annual appointment with my orthopedic surgeon, during which he took x-rays and measured for any variance in spinal curvature. Each year I watched with baited breath to find out if I was worse than the year before, knowing that if my scoliosis worsened, I would either be put in a body brace or have to undergo surgery to straighten my spine, neither of which sounded like an acceptable option. At around age twenty-four, I had my first "back attack." I bent over to pick up a piece of lint and my back seized into such a spasm that I couldn't breathe. I could hardly move and I was terrified. I didn't know what to do. At that time, following my doctor's advice, I opted for prescription painkillers.

My back spasms continued periodically throughout my twenties and thirties. The pain started on my lower left side and eventually seized the muscles around my ribcage. My doctor continued to recommend bedrest until the muscles let go, and muscle relaxants as needed. After a spasm occurred, I often just lay there, unable to move much because of the pain, feeling my heart slow down from the muscle relaxants, wondering if these medications were such a good idea. Sometimes the pain was so intense that I couldn't walk and found I needed to crawl about. These episodes, typically lasting three–

five days, left me fearing I could be in a wheelchair by age forty.

In my mid-twenties, I consulted a new doctor, an osteopath, who thought that I might find some relief from intense physical therapy. For two months, I attended physical therapy twice each week. Ultrasound provided no relief, nor did the exercises that I practiced religiously help at all. The only relief was from the stretching machine, where my shoulders and hips were strapped in and my body literally pulled apart. That felt good, but the pain returned once I was back up and about. I remember leaving physical therapy feeling better, getting in the car and driving forty-five miles to work, and barely being able to pull myself out of the car upon arriving at work. It then took several hours before I was able to stand up straight.

My painful back episodes were unpredictable. Just as the pain occurred, it all of a sudden disappeared, sometimes for several months. But, it always came back.

In my early thirties, I started managing my company's trade show program, with much travel involved, along with booth installation and dismantling. One day, while on one of these trips, I was standing in front of a mirror in my hotel room, putting on makeup. I felt a pain develop in my back and watched as my left hip started raising up, until it was visibly two–three inches higher than the right hip. The image I saw in the mirror was a deformed body. Even with my hips way out of alignment, I still had to go on, standing for most of the day. By the end of the day I was beside myself with pain and exhaustion. At this stage of my life, I had decided to steer clear of muscle relaxants and resigned myself to life with intermittent periods of intense pain.

I entered into a new phase of problems. My husband and I were redoing our front and backyard landscape and one afternoon I noticed that the outside of my left thigh developed numbness, such that I couldn't feel the fabric of my sweatpants against my skin. It was strange. I felt no pain, no tingling, no redness, no swelling, just surface numbness. I didn't even feel any back pain. I consulted my doctor, who saw no sign of neurological dysfunction. I was prescribed 100 mg of Norflex, to be taken over the next two weeks. Howering over me was my doctor's advice that I see an orthopedic surgeon if the numbness failed to clear up in four–six weeks.

Three days following this appointment, on a friend's advice, I consulted a Hanna somatic educator for the first time. She looked at my posture and took my history. She explained that my scoliosis was likely a functional (and thus fully resolvable) issue versus one of a structural nature. I was shocked. She also told me that I did not have a shorter left leg, that my scoliosis had my entire trunk off balance and that, once it was corrected, I would never again need to wear a lift in my shoe. At first, I thought I was hearing the ravings of a quack. Then she told me she thought we could resolve my scoliosis during the first one-hour session. I told her I didn't believe that was possible. So, she took a black marker and marked the vertebrae for a before and after comparison of my back. The markers clearly illustrated my "S" curve. She guided me in systematically de-contracting all the small muscles which attach the individual vertebrae to the large muscle groups. Afterward, and to my amazement, I looked in the mirror and saw that my "S" curve was no longer there. My spine was perfectly aligned! It felt like a miracle. And the whole process of our session was entirely pain free. In follow-up, she suggested two variations of an exercise (called Arch and Flatten) that I was to do twice daily to lengthen the muscles in my back and abdomen. She told me that I'd require at least several additional sessions before my range of issues was fully resolved.

During each of these sessions, as chronically tight muscles throughout my body released their grip, I felt a rush of heat energy flowing through that part of my body, almost like that area was awakening from a deep sleep. As a result of realigning my spine, eliminating my ribcage tilt, and aligning my hips and legs, I noticed that my clothes fit differently. I was able to wear one size smaller in jeans, as my real body shape was now somehow smaller. But, the biggest difference I felt was in the simple act of walking because I felt so much more at ease in my own body. In fact, I recall after my first session, going down to the beach and just enjoying the sensation of strolling along. My hips and entire trunk were loose; I felt like I was walking on air. Within two weeks of my first session, the numbness in my leg completely disappeared. I even felt my overall mood change. I felt happier and didn't find myself worrying as much. I found that I no longer woke up in the middle of the night needing to relieve myself.

In total, I had seven sessions with my Hanna somatic educator, five occurring over a period of four weeks, and two sessions about three months later. Besides the sessions, she prescribed a series of exercises for my particular vulnerable areas and suggested several Hanna somatic recorded exercise patterns that I should follow along to maintain my body. I found that there were particular exercises that I learned to do when I felt pain from overworking my body, such as the heavy-duty gardening work we were doing. If a pain developed in the lower left side of my back (my main trouble area), I would lie down and, in just a few minutes, easily free up that muscle group, then get up and be as good as new. To finally have control over my muscles was a dream come true."

Conditions and Indications

Somatics may provide substantial relief (if not outright resolve) from any condition that is caused, abetted, or complicated by sensorimotor amnesia. I repeat, somatic education is a neuromuscular modality, and as such may not be the preferred therapy for conditions involving primarily body systems other than the voluntary muscular (motor) system. That said, for every reason to not consider somatics, there are probably several favoring its use.

The following is a partial list of conditions for which somatic education may prove helpful: arthritis, back pain, balance problems, constrained breathing, carpal tunnel syndrome, constipation, fibromyalgia, foot pain, frequent urination, frozen parts, generalized stress, headaches (tension or sinus), hip pain, impotence, insomnia, joint pain, knee pain, neck pain, rotator cuff, sleeplessness, sacroiliac pain, sciatica, scoliosis, shoulder pain, spinal stenosis, spasms and cramps, sprains and strains, tennis elbow, thoracic outlet syndrome (TOS),

TMJ syndrome, torticollis, uneven leg length, whiplash, and more.

Even in cases of conditions for which HSE might not be indicated as a primary modality, non-muscular conditions often have neuromuscular concomitants, or "complications," as illustrated by several of the cases cited. Therefore, somatics should never be far from the forefront of consideration in any case of compromised health.

CHAPTER 9

CHILDREN AND SOMATICS

Nowhere is the saying "Why fix it if it ain't broke?" less apropos than in reference to children and their bodies. Preventative intervention can ensure that developing bodies are not subsequently saddled with the burdensome archeology of insults that weigh on most adults as they age. Early on in life is the ideal time to introduce healthy habits and preventive measures to avoid poor posture and flawed carriage later on. Plus, because young bodies haven't been around so long as to accumulate the usual stresses and tensions ensuing from a life lived, kids' bodies tend to be even more amenable to change than those of adults when fixing problems that have occurred.

Case 1. Adam, age twelve, was sullen and in obvious distress following a particularly traumatic afternoon of wrestling and trampoline jumping with older kids in the neighborhood. The very fact that he, usually stoic, complained at all convinced me he was in rough shape. Looking at the first photo [Figure 9-1a] note what appears to be a perfectly ordinary-looking boy. Only by comparison with the after photo [Figure 9-1b] can we recognize Adam's sunken chest and rounded shoulders in the previous photo. Those features, along with his sagging chin and pronounced lower back curvature, hint at the distress he was in before his session. One Lesson 2 Trauma reflex session was sufficient to mend his slumped and splinted posture and get him back to his usual perky self.

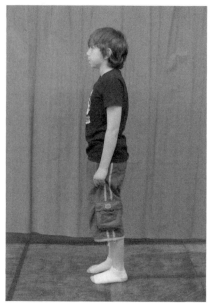
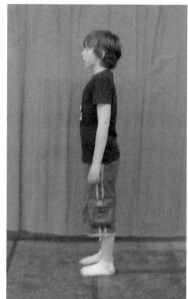

Figure 9-1a.   Figure 9-1b.

Naturally, there are some special considerations that need to be factored in when working with juveniles, especially younger kids. Much of the efficacy of somatics, as I've explained, is premised on self-sensing and the ability to introspect to differentiate muscular functions at a very fine level of control. For most younger kids, detailed or extended attention to self-sensing is just not a reasonable or realistic expectation. Childhood is about directing attention (sensing and experiencing) externally to the world outside, not the world within. Granted, children can have vivid imaginations and active fantasy lives, but these dynamics are substantively different from disciplined introspection. The upshot is most children have little interest or motivation, let alone ability, when it comes to matters of disciplined mindful attention to internal processes.

In my clinical setting, when I have a child on my table for this problem or that, I need to adjust my expectations and my language accordingly. For example, with adults I may get good mileage from my "dimmer switch" analogy in asking them to fine tune muscle contractions and releases. But not all kids are able to conceptualize such an abstract concept, even though they might already be familiar with how a dimmer switch works. I find it helps to keep an actual dimmer switch on hand that older youngsters can hold and feel, and practice with in order to role play how their bodies will perform. In theory at least, it becomes an easier matter to invoke a more concrete model as I ask them to contract or release certain muscles in a slow and controlled manner, just like the dimmer switch in their hands.

Occasionally, though, even this approach proves too abstract for youngsters. When faced with this obstacle I use a simple counting strategy—three counts to tighten a muscle so that youngsters learn to recruit muscles in a controlled and incremental fashion without jerking, and three counts to fully release the muscle(s) after tightening. This approach can be used with any child old enough to count. It's also helpful when working with kids to model for them, with their own bodies, the movements or positions I want them to assume. Whereas with adults it may be perfectly reasonable to expect them to raise their right shoulder toward their right ear when asked to do so, with kids it's best to move their shoulder for them toward their ear (this being an example of means whereby) to demonstrate first before asking them to follow suit on their own. Yet another helpful approach in getting kids to comport themselves in a somatic manner is to invoke an idealized character. Children, not otherwise inclined to organize or control their bodies as per a provider's agenda, can become remarkably compliant when imaging themselves performing as their favorite media hero, fictional or real.

Because children's bodies are usually so amenable to change, they may not need the same emphasis on home patterns as adults. In cases where patterns are indicated for home practice, things can be a little trickier with children. Kids naturally respond to the most interesting stimuli, so any patterns assigned need to be simple enough that kids are able to learn them. Also, the experience of doing the patterns needs to be entertaining enough ("entertaining" can mean fun or otherwise engaging of their attention, as long as it doesn't mean tedious or boring) to ensure compliance at home practice. The younger a child is, the less emphasis I place on introspection, personal process, or the like. Kids' brains are simply not wired for introspection, nor as capable of delayed gratification as adult brains. Kids would much rather have fun than engage in anything perceived as work. So, for kids, such patterns can be fashioned into games or even self contests ("...can you make your body look like an 'X'?...Now see if you can make this part of the 'X' longer," or "Move your back up and down like a slow-motion inchworm.").

If parents stay to observe their child's session I find it helpful to teach the patterns to parent and child both, so they can practice at home together. It never hurts to get the parents also experimenting with somatics movements. Aside from any direct benefits to parents, parental participation affords parents their own first-person experience at somatics. This can be helpful, first, as parents serve as natural role models for their children. When parents lead, kids may be more naturally inclined to follow suit. Second, in cases where children may be negligent or resistant to home practice, parents having had their own direct experience at movement patterns will have a basis for constructing helpful stories or narratives to reinforce or inspire their children's compliance.

Below, I've highlighted the case of a youngster I worked with to illustrate how significant changes in posture, carriage, and body mechanics can occur even at a young age.

Case 2. This is the case of a young boy, Dan, whose mother brought him in, reporting that his gait was off during running activities, so much so that he complained regularly of pain in his feet and had even begun avoiding games that called for running. He'd been in physical therapy for almost a year with negligible improvement. Given that the family placed a high value on sports and fitness, his discomfort at running was perceived as problematic, more so than might have been the case had the child been a bookworm or a musician rather than a budding athlete.

In the before and after photos below, observe the marked difference after just a first session. Before [Figure 9-2a], Dan's feet are closed and both turned slightly to his left. Relative to his lower body, the right side of his waist is pulled back, as is the entire right side of his back and shoulder area, and his head is turned slightly askew, to his left. In sum, his middle body goes one way, while his lower and uppermost body goes the other way, making for a clear case of Trauma posture.

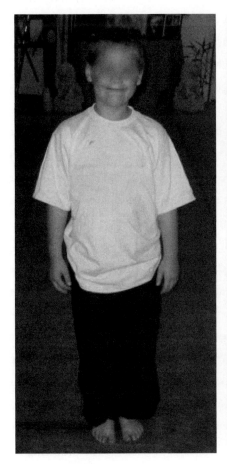 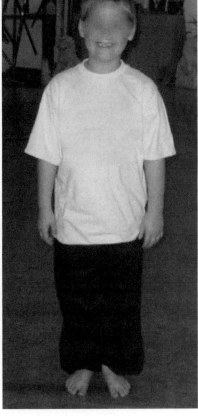

Figure 9-2a.   Figure 9-2b.

After a Lesson 2, Dan's feet, legs and torso, extending up through his shoulders, are nearly perfectly aligned [Figure 9-2b]. His head appears tilted left, yet it is centered (not turned) from the perspective of both ears being equally visible. I speculated that Dan's head might well right itself, vertically, as is often the case without further intervention. In fact, that is exactly what happened before a week passed. Had his head not righted itself, this would simply have become fodder for a second session. As it turned out, one session proved sufficient to correct Dan's issues and improve his gait while running.

Given how the effects of sensorimotor amnesia accumulate and compound due to an archeology of insults, it follows that the sooner one nips this process of decline in the bud the better. When better to start fixing a problem than earlier on, before it gains a solid foothold in the body?

These days young bodies incur a great deal more stress, and stress of a different kind as compared to earlier generations. Knapsacks and book bags are loaded heavier and make their debut in a child's life at an earlier age. Hours at a time may be spent hunched over a computer screen, or in front of video games or television. Cocking one's head to chat on the telephone is no longer something done just at home but has evolved into a lifestyle expression with the advent of cell phones that accompany kids everywhere they go. It's no wonder kids and their bodies are under so much duress these days.

Of the many unhealthy influences (stressors) around kids and adults, no single one can be implicated with any real certainly as the single, or even primary, identifiable cause of various health problems. These influences include, but are not limited to, air and water pollution; heavily sugared and artificially sweetened foods; various environmental toxins such as off-gassing from construction materials, printers, and copying machines; secondhand tobacco smoke, food preservatives and coloring agents; residues from food chain pesticides, antibiotics and growth hormones; violence and gratuitous sex in the media; the pressures of increasingly younger team sports; questionable vaccinations; carbonated beverages; high fat/low nutrient diets; medication side effects and iatrogenic illnesses; nutrient-poor fast or prepackaged foods; dysfunctional family dynamics, substance abuse, peer pressure, and bullying; indoor air quality; and last, but not least, electromagnetic pollution.[1] No doubt you can add to this list if you put your mind to it. Perhaps not all of these concerns apply in any individual case; but several of them, at least, apply in every case. Any and all of these are tantamount to insults such as I've discussed in earlier chapters. When considered according to their collective effect, these are issues and concerns that stress bodies both directly and indirectly and compromise people's resilience in withstanding other more physiologic stressors. It is also a matter of no small concern that any or all of these toxic influences exert a different and more pronounced effect on the developing bodies and brains of children than they do on fully mature adults.[2]

Despite the pervasive presence of these various health dangers in our society, I have yet to see any scientific, corporate/industrial or governmental authority performing metastudies to comprehensively examine how contributions from multiple sources add up to a dangerous whole in determining the cumulative effects of these toxic influences on our children. Surely, the total effect must be greater than the sum of the individual parts. Where are our social priorities and accountabilities that we expose our children to these (in many cases, scientifically proven) dangers? Happily, and remarkably, the developing human body appears very forgiving and extraordinarily resilient. Even so, the developing bodies of children need all the help they can get; and the sooner and younger that help is available to them the better. Somatics can at least serve to minimize the effects of muscular and postural stress.

Recall the first client cited in this chapter. Exactly one year subsequent to his earlier circumstance, Adam (again in typical teenage fashion) wrought havoc on his body, this time stemming from a combination of skateboarding, rough play, and growth spurt. He came to me complaining of back pain. His middle and upper back area was taut; both arms and shoulders were visibly

---

1 According to Andrew Weil, M.D. (See *Spontaneous Healing*), "...electromagnetic pollution may be the most significant form of pollution human activity has produced in this century, all the more dangerous because it is invisible and insensible."
2 Jordana Miller, "Tests reveal high chemical levels in kids' bodies," CNN. 10/22/07.

rotated outward and retracted back. His right-side leg and waist were also retracted [Figure 9-3a]. As with his earlier circumstance a single somatics session worked wonders for his posture [Figure 9-3b] and substantially relieved his back pain. This serves to underscore the value of somatics as an ongoing resource for developing bodies—for nipping problems in the bud, so to speak—before they become firmly established as pathological reflex patterns.

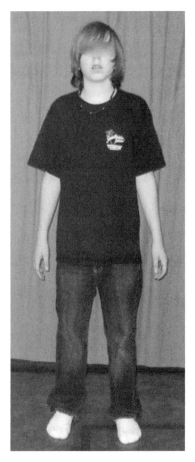 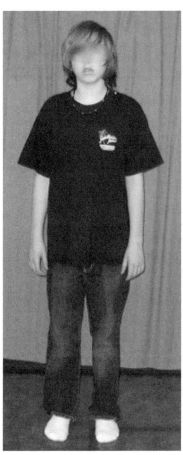

Figure 9-3a.   Figure 9-3b.

Insults: How They Occur and How Their Effects Accumulate

Let's take a look here at how some specific insults might occur, starting at a young age, and how their effects accumulate, compounding the toll they take on the body (or indeed on the whole person) over time. Keep in mind that these are simplified scenarios.

Scenario #1

Some insults can be perpetrated against the body as a result of enculturation and social values. A perfect example of this can be seen in the way girls are singled out for gender roles as different from boys. Let's take just a cursory look at a single decade in the life of Alice. Naturally, the following scenario doesn't apply to all girls, but many who read this will recognize familiar themes and circumstances.

From the time girls are quite young, and according to the values of their parents, teachers, and other role models, they are often taught to "protect" themselves by concealing and not revealing, to remain "ladylike." From early on, girls may be instructed in the niceties of crossing their legs when they sit in a skirt, so as not to overexpose. Even in cases where parents are not heavy-handed about this, the tacit message may be that there is something to hide, protect, or be ashamed of. Combine this parochial message with Alice's personality, which is already shy and reticent, and the message and her natural predisposition combine to become mutually reinforcing dynamics. Alice is one of those children who seems unduly self-conscious from the time she can walk and talk. Throughout childhood her demeanor is quiet, she always crosses her legs tightly when sitting, and avoids drawing attention to herself. As a young adolescent Alice hits puberty and her womanly features begin to develop. Her response is to shrink away from the kind of attention engendered by that same development in her peers who are learning to deal with, and even enjoying, attention from male classmates. Alice wants none of that. More than a little self-conscious now, she feels somewhat ashamed of herself for succumbing to nature's course. She wears unflattering sweaters and hunches her shoulders forward. Her posture fully reflects, and now even exaggerates, her shy demeanor. She has retreated into herself. Her posture also affects the regard with which her teachers and other adults hold her, so that academically, as well as socially, she is left to slip between the cracks. Nobody expects much from such a retiring young girl. Meanwhile, she still has to lug around her heavy backpack of textbooks, adding further stress to her body and exacerbating her tendency to lean forward. Consequently, along with hunching her shoulders Alice is beginning to lean from her middle and lower back. By junior high school she is evidencing a marked kyphosis,[3] the first indication of what, forty or fifty years hence, will likely be regarded in her as a dowager's hump. And, because she has spent her whole life crossing her legs due to reasons she never quite fathomed, her adductor and internal rotator muscles have become habituated to that role. As a result, Alice's gait is short and tentative, precluding any natural swing in her hips.

Obviously, I could continue to build on this story. Just as clearly, Alice could benefit from more than just somatics in addressing her personal issues. But our immediate concern here is with Alice's body issues. This brief scenario gives you enough information to develop a basic appreciation of how body issues, in this case seen from their early stages of development, will have an important bearing on Alice's future, both in reflection and reinforcement of her own personal identity. So I ask you, where do you see Alice's body in another decade, or two, or three? How might her life have been different if not for her early indoctrination and the resulting habituated patterns?

Scenario #2

Robert is a teenager who lives by the seashore. His great passion in life is music, and he shows real promise with several instruments, including drums,

---

3 Kyphosis is an exaggerated forward curvature of the upper back/neck, e.g., humpback.

harmonica, and his own personal favorite, the saxophone. Robert likes to hang out with his longtime best friend over weekends, and during summer vacation the two of them spend time exploring along the local coastline in their kayaks. One day, while kayaking, a stiff breeze kicks up and Robert's friend spills overboard. There's no real danger here as both are properly equipped with buoyancy vests and they're only in waist-deep water. However, as Robert struggles to stabilize his friend's craft until the other boy can get back on board, a strong gust, timed just wrong with a wave, sweeps the lighter empty kayak toward shore. Clutching to hold his friend's kayak steady, while trying to maintain the stability of his own craft against nature's force, proves too much for Robert's shoulder, causing the muscles of his shoulder and upper back to give way. Robert's family doctor puts him in an arm sling for several weeks, and that's that. An ordinary injury for an ordinary teenager dealt with in an ordinary manner.

Except that none of this proves ordinary for Robert. Once the sling comes off, Robert's shoulder continues to bother him. The pains are sharp and more than occasional, and his shoulder feels weaker and droops noticeably. Robert is forced to give up saxophone because his shoulder can no longer support the weight of this instrument for more than a few minutes without hurting, and his timing as a drummer suffers as well. Absenting the other instruments, the harmonica fails to satisfy Robert's musical urges and, without a great deal of thought to the matter, Robert gradually drifts away from music altogether.

With his departure from music, Robert's prospect of a full musical scholarship evaporates into thin air. He no longer has reason to keep up his circle of musical friends. He becomes disconsolate and his grades plummet. This makes Robert more despondent and he starts experimenting with drugs. A minor run-in with the law shakes up Robert a bit, but nothing really changes. After limping through high school he takes a job in sales, which entails a great deal of travel. Occasionally his job calls for heavy lifting, which aggravates his old shoulder injury. Robert never gets back on track with his music.

How much fulfillment is Robert likely to experience as his life unfolds?

How might his life have been different had his musical career blossomed? And, is that shoulder likely to get better, or worse?

Scenario #3

Bobby's father is in sales, so every year or two the family relocates to a new area. Bobby hates picking up and leaving his friends and familiar environment for new digs. Every new area has a different set of social norms, which Bobby isn't too keen on. He figures out early on, though, that athletic abilities are the key to making friends and earning respect fast, so he becomes adept at sports. His most recent relocation, however, has offered up a new challenge in bullies at school. Fortunately, a martial arts academy is close at hand and Bobby decides to try it out. As it turns out, martial arts not only provide a solution to Bobby's bully problem but elicit in him a new passion. He feels a developing sense of power and autonomy as he keeps up his training over the years, the very opposite of the disempowerment he felt each time his parents decided to uproot and relocate. This new passion also presents ample opportunities for bumps, bruises, strains, and fractures as Bob, now a young man, assumes the helm of his school with his teacher's retirement. The physical demands of teaching are relentless, but Bob loves the challenge. He pushes his body with strength-building exercises, speed-building techniques, and stretching until his body totters at his limits, and sometimes beyond. As the years go by, the litany of injuries begins to take its toll. Stiffness appears where previously there'd been flexibility, caution where there'd been abandon, and an assortment of therapies to treat that pesky neck and back that keep "going out" where formerly there'd been only youthful vigor.

Where do you think Bob might at be today with that declining body of his? How long do you think he can he keep up this pace at his chosen career before the demands on his body become too great?

In Summary

I composed these three scenarios because they demonstrate how sensorimotor amnesia can be rooted in early and formative experiences, and how it is that different and varied experiences (physical, social, emotional, intrinsic, extrinsic) can all come to bear in their collective impact on the physical body in a complicated and burdensome archeology. In each case, somatics might have been, or might still be, introduced at any stage to mitigate the effects of these insults and the trajectory of decline they portend. These accounts leave me musing over how helpful early intervention with somatics might have been had it been available and opted for at an early age. Somatics is perfectly safe for kids, and could probably be introduced even as early as six to ten years of age, when it could spare youngsters, and adults-to-be, a lifetime of unnecessary pain and suffering.

Somatic education is primarily a physical modality. It addresses errant sensorimotor patterns as they occur in the body. You must keep in mind, however, that the body is not always just the body. In many cases, physical trauma or decline, such as are implicated in sensorimotor amnesia, can have a profound effect on one's personal psychology, attitude, and outlook on life. In the interests of optimal wellness and achieving your own human potential, remain mindful that your body, your mind, and your spirit exist as different—but not as separate and unconnected—aspects of your "self." This is every bit as true for children as it is for adults.

PART 3

MUSINGS, ESSAYS, QUESTIONS, AND ANSWERS

The Chapters in Part 3 represent a compilation of essays, lectures and Q & A covering a diverse range of topics concerning somatics. Be forewarned: this is a mix of reputable science, conjecture, theory, and pure opinion. I expect some of these perspectives to be useful, and some even provocative (hopefully in a good way).

CHAPTER 10

MUSINGS AND SUCH

The Importance of Deep Abdominal Breathing to Your Health

The all too common tendency to breathe in a manner that is shallow, or constrained, is one of the great banes of modern man. Habitual shallow chest breathing is a major precursor for cardiovascular problems and respiratory problems, as well as a host of other health issues. That this particular problem is so endemic in modern society is no coincidence. Shallow breathing is both a cause and a reflection of many health problems.

Two of the most common causes of shallow breathing[1] are a tight gut and chronic low grade stress, both of which are more often attributable to lifestyle causes than to bone fide medical conditions. Ironically, flat bellies and tight guts are much sought after in society by men and women alike. The media promotes the virtues of a flat belly relentlessly, and popular approaches to exercise and fitness regularly invoke flat bellies and tight guts as the prevailing measures of their success. Nevertheless, flat guts, and especially the means by which they are accomplished, are of dubious value. Flat bellies are, in and of themselves, fine and harmless; but when they are achieved by measures that contribute to chronic tightness in the muscles of the abdomen (or elsewhere), they become dangerous.

Our second precursor, chronic low-grade stress, can be attributed to a wide range of causes. Chronic stress often causes the body's sympathetic nervous trigger to become stuck in the "on" position, effectively precluding the body's ability to stand down and relax. These concerns—tightness of the gut and low-grade stress—are but two of many component parts in a self-fulfill-

---

1 Smoking is so obvious it doesn't warrant mention here.

ing health risk syndrome comprising a neurophysiological cycle.

The thoracic diaphragm, which attaches at its perimeter along the inner rim of the lower ribcage, is the primary muscle responsible for controlling breath. The diaphragm is a vaulted muscle when it is relaxed, shaped roughly like an open umbrella, or mushroom cap. The diaphragm causes us to inhale by contracting down flat toward the abdomen to create a vacuum pressure in the lungs, this in much the same manner as a fireplace bellows that must be inflated before it can be squeezed shut. The more efficiently the diaphragm is able to contract, the more efficiently air will be drawn into the lungs. But, like a bellows that fails to open all the way, the diaphragm can only draw breath into the lungs according to its freedom to function properly in an unrestricted manner. If the diaphragm can't contract fully, we can't breathe fully.

Most people, even seasoned athletes, breathe well below one hundred percent efficiency. In fact, the average person uses considerably less than twenty-five percent of their actual lung capacity during normal breathing.[2] In cases of chronic respiratory distress, tidal volume[3] at ten percent or less of total capacity is not at all uncommon. Granted, the lungs have a tremendous reserve capacity, which is to say that none of us needs to be breathing at, or even near, full capacity to procure all the oxygen we need under normal circumstances. Even so, the more fully we can breathe, the more easily we can oxygenate our many tissues to increase the overall efficiency of our respiratory process.

An important point to grasp is that constrained breathing is but one part of a cyclical problem. As is often the case with cycles, once established there is no clearly identifiable starting point for this pattern. For one person, constrained breathing might start with emotional anxiety or depression or stress, while for another it might stem from improper exercise in a quest to develop six-pack abs. The cultural preoccupation with achieving a flat belly by any means certainly doesn't contribute to healthy breathing. Even factors outside one's control, e.g., environmental pollutants such as might occur due to

---

2 As per personal correspondence with Bill Stenson M.D., pulmonologist.

3 (aka T.V.), The amount of air breathed in or out during normal respiration.

smog, mining conditions, wildfires, home projects, or off-gassing from common chemical sources, can be implicated in constrained breathing patterns.

The thoracic diaphragm, in order to contract down flat, must be able to shift the viscera (organs and such) downward and out of the way to make room for itself as it contracts, which explains why deep abdominal breathing causes your belly to expand forward on inhalation. A hypothetical trigger for constrained breathing might occur when someone hears upsetting news that creates emotional anxiety. This, or any other chronic or acute stressor, can automatically excite the body's sympathetic (fight or flight) nervous response with a resultant tightness in the muscles of the gut.

If tightness in the gut muscles lock up the viscera, the diaphragm has less room to contract. You can easily experience this yourself if you tighten your gut [pause here to try this now] and try to take in a deep breath. Notice your limited capacity for breath intake. The tightness in your gut creates an actual physical impediment that prevents the diaphragm from contracting down flat to open the lungs fully. Meanwhile, this same tightness tends to exert a downward pulling force on the ribcage, further impeding respiratory function by effectively preventing the ribs from expanding naturally with the intake of breath. Tightness such as this, when chronic, results in habitually short and inefficient breaths.

Any number of seemingly benign stimuli can elicit a tight gut reaction. Imagine the following scenario while you press your fingers firmly into your abdomen: you're driving a car and a ball or small animal appears suddenly in your path. As you instinctively reach with your foot for the brake pedal, feel how your gut tightens automatically. I can only imagine how taxing it must be on respiratory efficiency for individuals who commute regularly in heavy traffic. Myriad stressors occurring every day, and repeatedly eliciting a tight gut response, can contribute to habituation of this same response so that reflexive tightness in your gut, rather than a relaxed belly, becomes your norm. This makes for a classic case of Red Light reflex syndrome.

The greatest risk of chronic tightness in the gut is falling into the habit of shallow breathing. Even when breathing inefficiently, the body's cardiovascular demands remain constant. The heart must continuously pump oxygen-rich blood throughout the body. In compensation for less oxygen being available due to constrained breathing patterns, the body may employ any or all of several compensatory responses. First, red blood cell production may increase to deliver more oxygen to the capillaries. However, too many additional red blood cells will thicken the blood (absolute polycythemia), eliciting a hyperventilatory response, meaning the heart must beat both faster to make up for less efficient oxygenation of the blood, and harder to pump blood that is now more viscous.

Shallow breathing, combined with poor oxygenation, in turn raises blood pressure to service the ongoing needs of the body. This is the physiological equivalent of running a car's engine constantly in the Red zone, and places the body under tremendous duress. Not unreasonably, the brain's response to all of this is one of (exacerbated) chronic low-level anxiety. The cycle worsens as even low-level anxiety increases the oxygen demand while diminishing the ability to absorb oxygen efficiently. This can result in possible tendencies toward depression, short temper, impatience, disturbed sleep patterns, digestive difficulties, etc. Additionally, the mechanics of shallow breathing undermine the syphoning of lymph from the thoracic duct. Last, but not least, constrained breathing can cause fatigue, both mental and physical, as well as reduced stamina.

The brain consumes approximately twenty-five percent of the oxygen you inhale. When oxygen becomes less available to the whole body due to constrained breathing, the brain experiences the effects of oxygen deprivation just like the rest of the body. Even healthy breathers expend approximately five percent of their energy just on the process of breathing. Individuals whose breathing is severely compromised, as in extreme cases like emphysema, may expend up to fifty percent of their total body energy, day and night, on breathing alone![4]

---

4 Ruth Werner, *A Massage Therapist's Guide to Pathology*, 3rd Edition. Lippincott, Williams, & Wilkins, 2005.

Any or all of these symptoms can reflect and/or reinforce the body's chemical and hormonal imbalance, causing serotonin levels to decrease and cortisol (a major stress hormone) to increase, further complicating this debilitating cycle. Even just simple generalized anxiety perpetuates this cycle by alarming the sympathetic nervous system and reinforcing any tendency to breathe shallowly. Oh, and I almost forgot—reduced oxygen intake puts one of your primary memory areas at risk as well with a double whammy. The hippocampus is vulnerable both to the aforementioned increased levels of cortisol, and extremely sensitive to the reduced oxygen levels[5] that result from shallow and constrained breathing.

What can you do about this and why should you act? Somehow this cycle must be broken in order for the body and all of its systems—cardiovascular, nervous, endocrine, digestive, lymphatic, etc.—to stand down and relax to a level of normal healthy functioning. Barring this normality, one may fully expect all the effects of a stressed-out system to ensue. It is merely a question of when, and of which part of your system breaks down first under duress—your heart, your anxiety level/mood, your vascular function, your digestion/elimination, your respiratory system, or some other chronic illness. Take your pick.

You can take steps to interrupt this cycle at any point. The easiest way to enact self-intervention is to learn how to relax your breath and breathe fully in an abdominal fashion. The very act of paying attention to how you breathe represents a first step in reversing this debilitating process. A firmly entrenched pattern of shallow breathing will also benefit from participation at Tai Chi or somatics, or in some cases yoga. Both these methods offer useful and direct measures for helping you learn how to relax and breathe in a manner that will make deep abdominal breathing the habit that it should be.

The somatics breathing patterns included in Thomas Hanna's *The Myth of Aging* series, and expanded upon in his *Full Breathing* series, are the most effective I have encountered at interrupting this cycle to restore an internal environment conducive to deep abdominal breathing. By my way of thinking,

---

5 Louis Cozolino, *The Healthy Aging Brain*. Norton, 2008.

these particular breathing patterns should serve as a basis for anyone involved in disciplines that emphasize breath work, including qigong, martial arts, yoga, and singing. Taijiquan (or yoga), when properly practiced, becomes an excellent means of reinforcing deep breathing patterns on an ongoing basis. Get started today.

Abandonment

Ever since the fateful words, "...why hast thou forsaken me?" were uttered so very long ago, abandonment has been relegated near-mortal-sin status. In more modern times issues such as spousal abandonment, along with the even worse "child abandonment," have raised eyebrows. The armed forces have their own acronym, AWOL (absent without leave), to describe abandonment specific to their genre. Always, abandonment carries with it the connotation of futility, negligence, or desperation in the face of a lost cause.

Sometimes, however, abandonment can be more benign, as when it results from plain and simple neglect, such as an abandoned car, an abandoned friendship, or "that old abandoned barn out back." This distinction may be of small consequence to whatever or whomever has been abandoned. But, for the perpetrator, this distinction offers the prospect of some reprieve—stop abandoning and the effects of the neglect may be reversed.

Less dramatic than our initial examples above, but still to the point, are the ways in which abandoner and abandonee can be one and the same. Oh yes, we can abandon ourselves. We can do so according to complex psychological or spiritual dispositions by shutting down emotions or by living our lives in denial. Or, we can do so with our bodies in ways that hardly draw attention. In fact, sensorimotor amnesia (SMA) such as is addressed in somatic education is unquestionably the most pandemic form of abandonment known to humankind. Sensorimotor amnesia might as well be called sensorimotor abandonment, because during this state of affairs the brain has, de facto, abandoned a part or parts of the body.

However, because sensorimotor amnesia is often subtle, both in its on-set and its appearance, it is poorly recognized. This also renders it insidious. Due to the nature of SMA, few who suffer from this form of abandonment even know that they suffer, let alone from what they suffer. At least this is usually the case early on. These sufferers are the unwitting victims of their own neglect. Sensorimotor amnesia presents itself in such a variety of simple guises that even modern medicine with all its technological resources fails to recognize SMA for what it is.

Instead of seeing sensorimotor amnesia, modern science and medicine sees only its effects: arthritis, various and sundry pain syndromes, postural decline, and the most ubiquitously ignorant mislabeling of all—just getting older. Not that arthritis or pain syndromes can't be bone fide indications of declining health, but much more often than conventional medicine is aware these conditions either are caused by or are abetted by sensorimotor amnesia. As such, these conditions are often amenable to change once the abandon-ment has been redressed.

As a martial arts teacher, I regularly witness abandonment in Kung Fu and Tai Chi students as well. This is a matter of particular concern with Tai Chi because such abandonment is antithetical to Tai Chi's most basic tenets. This shortcoming can be observed when any part of the body, or movement of said part, fails to function according to the practitioner's clear and deliber-ate intention. In Tai Chi this may be seen, typically, when a student's atten-tion misses the gestalt and falls disproportionately on the leg that is stepping, or the arm or hand that seems most to be leading a movement, whilst the more passive leg or arm (or other body part) is at least temporarily abandoned to a less prominent and less fully integrated role. Granted, this may fall well short of mortal sin status for most folks. But in the context of a discipline in which movements are sought to be deliberate and precisely controlled even to a level of nuance, abandonment would seem to stall one at cross purposes. Conversely, as students gradually over time (or perhaps more expediently through the practice of somatics) improve their self-sensing abilities, so will they relinquish the tendency to abandon in favor of more fully integrated and differentiated movement.

In non-Tai Chi scenarios, abandonment can readily be seen in individuals displaying habituated reflex patterns. In such circumstances muscles or muscles groups fail to relax completely when the brain is not actively calling them into service, the consequence being that muscles become stuck to some degree or other in chronic contraction. The brain then, by default, turns its attention to those parts of the body that still fall under its voluntary control. This creates a quandary as any muscle saddled with any degree of stuckness, or hypertonus, is immediately cast in conflict with its antagonist muscles, muscles with which there would ordinarily exist a relative détente. You need only glance around at others to observe such scenarios, though noting for compromised postures in others may take some practice.

Because of the prevalence in our society of SMA, we've become desensitized such that we rarely attach importance to habituated patterns as conditions of note. We may notice the pronounced limp, but rarely the raised shoulder or the lordotic back. When postural dissonance is the rule rather than the exception, there is scant reason for it to catch our attention. Even when we do notice such issues they are usually attributed to just getting older.

Fortunately, the prospect of reprieve, at least from neuromuscular abandonment, is readily at hand. Thanks to the legacy of Thomas Hanna we have the means by which sensorimotor amnesia and abandonment issues can be largely eliminated. Hanna's many dozens of movement patterns and hands-on techniques—assisted pandiculation foremost among them—can quickly and easily redress neuromuscular abandonment that is due to sensorimotor amnesia. HSE movement patterns and table work are uniquely effective in restoring full voluntary control by teaching clients to pay attention to differentiate muscle functions and behaviors, thereby reclaiming them from the realm of amnesia or reflex. The simple act of paying attention in a discerning manner already improves awareness and control where previously there was abandonment.

Repeatedly, I have heard my own personal initial reactions to this system of wellness restoration echoed in the words of others—"But how can it possibly work, it's SO simple." Indeed, how can something so simple, in a world accustomed to seeking its answers in complex technologies, provide such an effective and comprehensive solution to human pain and suffering as somatic education? No matter how advanced and complicated are the technologies we develop and live with, the simple fact remains that our own bodies have not evolved on a par with technology. The human body is essentially the same as it's been for tens of thousands of years—the same muscles, the same brain, and the same tolerances for use and abuse. The low tech principles of somatics could as easily have been discovered during the Middle Ages as now, so elementary to the human condition are its methods and basic tenets. And now, as then, reversing the effects of sensorimotor amnesia, aka abandonment, is as simple as insuring that your brain and the muscles of your motor system are communicating freely and effectively in the absence of impediments to doing so. Accomplish that and, *voila!*, no more abandonment.

Sex as an Insult (Can You Believe?)

At first blush, I wish I had some discreet spot where I could sequester this article as separate from the rest of my text so as not to offset what credibility I have gained with the reader thus far. The commentary and opinions that follow are bound to be perceived as controversial by some, but sex—at least the wrong kind of sex—is an insult I cannot ignore. Keep in mind; I'm not talking about insulting sex. That's an altogether different topic.

There are certain primitive drives that govern behavior across the animal kingdom, regardless of how advanced or, in the case of humans, how civilized a species may be. For humans, these drives include sustenance from food and water, thermal stability (keeping warm and dry) sufficient to maintain homeostasis, and the drive to reproduce. These several drives pretty much sum up nature's agenda for us humans. My focus here is on the latter of these drives. All species procreate, and some even rely on sex as a "political platform" from which to maintain control within the natural pecking order. A rare few (primate) species have even been observed to engage in recreational sex. By comparison, humans have taken their expression of sex to levels of artistically creative and recreational divergence not seen elsewhere in the animal kingdom. Humans are perfectly capable of being spurred in their sexual behavior by ulterior motives and artifice, as well as by cultural or social mandates. In short, sex for humans is often about much more than sex. And even when sex is about sex it may have nothing whatsoever to do with procreation.

My point in all this is that while the sex drive can be powerful, even urgent, and unquestionably delightful at times, it can also be quite unreasonable. And unreasonable behavior, especially when coupled with powerful natural urges, can easily result in unintended consequences. The powerful and rhythmic thrusting motions that often characterize sexual intercourse typically assume primacy over all other body functions and concerns while the sex act is in progress, and may even rival the rigors of competitive sports in their demands on the body.[6] The greater part of this exertion centers at the body's midsection, in the hips, waist, and lower back.[7] Other athletes and fitness aficionados warm up and stretch out before vigorous activity to minimize the likelihood of bodily injury, but not so with the average person (pardon my assumption) prior to sex. At best, most lovers-to-be probably engage in foreplay. In my opinion, sex that is overly vigorous or overly frequent puts

---

6 This is a stereotype not applicable to all persons always.

7 This can certainly be the case for persons not educated in more spiritually evolved methods of sexual expression. There are traditions of sexual expression stemming from Tantra or Taoist alchemy, to name two that I'm aware of, for which the culmination of sexual release is not a primary goal. Rather, these practices promote more *process oriented* methods of sexual expression that could easily be converted to HSE-like exercises within the context of sexual union. For example, from a strictly mechanical perspective, the aforementioned thrusting movements characteristic of missionary sex are nothing more than a variant on the somatics pattern known as Arch and Flatten in their alternating engagement of the powerful muscles of the lower back and of the abdomen. The somatics pattern is slow, mindful, and methodical, not to mention solo and non-sexual, while its more sexual counterpart is typically one of urgent abandon rooted in carnal instinct. Notably, any movement or motor function that is mindless can be brought to the conscious fore in a more conscientious fashion to alter one's experience, ala Tantric or Taoist alchemy. This approach could offer people who are limited in their ability for sexual expression, due for example to back pain, a whole new range of possibilities, perhaps even akin to what Viagra, et. al., has made possible for those suffering from erectile dysfunction.

both parties at risk, and men more so than women. Men are more at risk, not only because they tend to be more aggressive in their exertions (I apologize in advance to those exceptions to this stereotype), but because they ejaculate. According to the precepts of traditional Chinese medicine (TCM), sexual excess depletes kidney jing.[8] Even here in the West there is a basis for this belief in folk wisdom (recall Burgess Meredith's famous line from the movie *Rocky*, "Women weaken legs." You'll recall, also, that the kidneys are positioned in close proximity to the lower back. When the kidney jing becomes deficient the low back, waist area and hips, as well as the Wei Qi[9] function suffer the consequences. Sexual excess, excess being the operative word, can thus be a precursor to, if not a direct cause of low back pain, stiffness, and more.

In Chapter 5, I described how our fictional character, Joe, suffered from a concomitant loss of virility as a result of sensorimotor amnesia that stemmed from a seemingly unrelated injury. I also described how somatics, albeit inadvertently, helped him to regain that virility by undoing the causes for its loss. I suspect that quite a few men suffering from low back pain also happen to suffer from diminished libido (as separate from any aversion to sex caused by back pain), which may be caused or abetted, ironically, by sexual overindulgence.

Let's look at some figures for both back pain and erectile dysfunction data to get a sense of the scope of these respective problems. It is estimated that more than eighty percent of all adults will experience at least an episode of lower back pain at some point in their lives[10], and many individuals live

---

8 *Jing* is the term used in traditional Chinese medicine to describe procreative, or sexual, energy. Jing is stored in the kidneys and is understood to govern the bones, as well as the reproductive function. Depleted jing weakens the constitution overall. Men are understood to deplete jing via ejaculation, women more so via menstruation and childbirth.

9 *Wei Qi* is regarded as the body's first line of defense against illness and injury. Wei Qi acts like a bubble pack, or force field, to mitigate the effects of physical trauma. A strong Wei Qi function also bolsters the body's immune system against certain pathogens (evil and pernicious influences ala TCM) and other stressors.

10 "'Alarming Increase' In Prevalence Of Chronic Low-Back Pain: UNC Study," Article dated 2/10/09. As per Timothy S. Carey, M.D., director of the Sheps Center in the UNC School of Medicine and Janet K. Freburger, Ph.D, research scientist at the UNC Institute on Aging. Accessed 10/1/10. http://www.medicalnewstoday.com/articles/138422.php.

with chronic back pain. Meanwhile, the Massachusetts study data suggests there will be approximately 617,715 new cases of erectile dysfunction in the United States annually.[11] Extrapolated across the study's thirty-year age allowance that calculates out to approximately eighteen million cases of erectile disorder, give or take a few, at any given time. That's a lot of back pain and a lot of erectile disorder. I surmise there is a good bit of overlap between the two. Of course, this correlation hardly amounts to a scientifically valid connection, but one certainly has to wonder at the prevalence of both back pain and erectile dysfunction (especially in light of TCM theory), and entertain the possibility that more than mere happenstance may be at work here. If you've not entertained the thought previously, you might now be musing whether there could be some connection between your lovemaking and your back pain. So, what to do?

Far be it for me to suggest that people stop engaging in sex to avoid its potential as an insult. However, too much or the wrong kind of sex can contribute just as easily as too much or the wrong kind of any other physically demanding activity to muscular habituation and sensorimotor amnesia with its plethora of symptoms. I suggest (in lieu of your opting for outright abstinence) that this may be one very important area in your life where the daily practice of somatic movement patterns can prove useful in offsetting the effects of those insults that would result in sensorimotor amnesia—insults that might otherwise rob you of your virility and your ability to engage freely in healthy sexual communication.

Somatics and Other Martial Arts

Martial artists, and especially martial arts teachers, ought to learn everything they can about somatic education at first opportunity. The advantages of both

---

11   C.B.Johannes, A.B. Araujo, H.A. Feldman, "Incidence of erectile dysfunction in men 40 to 69 years old: Longitudinal results from the Massachusetts Male Aging Study," *J Urol.* 163: 2000; 460-463. Accessed 10/1/10. http://www.clevelandclinicmeded.com/medicalpubs/diseasemanagement/endocrinology/erectile-dysfunction/.

direct hands-on HSE work and the only slightly more benign effects of so-matics movement patterns, such as those taught in *The Myth of Aging* series, as well as other series, make for compelling martial arts training adjuncts.

Aside from all the other intriguing reasons to experience somatics, HSE is a great way for teachers of martial arts (or any movement discipline) to mini-mize student loss due to injuries or physical limitations. Many of the injuries that do occur in martial arts schools are not caused by martial arts training, per se, but rather are triggered according to preexisting conditions (i.e., inju-ries waiting to happen). Somatics can nip these injuries in the bud by elimi-nating the predisposition before the injury occurs to sideline the student.

Martial arts are very much about maximizing aspects of human potential, and somatics promotes a level of body awareness and control that allows for the best kind of flexibility, leaving practitioners to feel more in control of their own bodies. While in the early stages of writing this book I had occasion to teach a "Myth of Aging" seminar at a martial arts school in another state. The twenty or so participants in attendance were so impressed that several unsolicited phone calls and emails attested to the impressive gains attendees made as a result of the seminar. Students expressed their gratitude that the HSE patterns had facilitated a whole range of new physical possibilities, all in just that one weekend. One student reported that he'd been passed over for his Black Belt test because his physical limitations rendered him ineligible. After that single "Myth of Aging" workshop he reported he no longer felt the same limitations. Another participant, the event host, offered that he felt tall-er after just the first several patterns taught on day one. At first, he'd chalked this up to his imagination, until he found he needed to readjust his car's rear view mirror before driving the next morning, due to his increased stature.

Somatics is also a great way to offer expanded service to existing clientele. Teachers who have received training as somatic educators[12] may have less cause, or need, to refer injured or impaired clients elsewhere for remedial services such as massage, chiropractic, or physical therapy once they themselves have the train-

---

12   See Resources in Chapter 17 for information on HSE practitioner training.

ing and skills necessary to help students recover, or to help their students avoid injuries in the first place. When students do report injuries, teachers trained in somatics can be better equipped to help them in a way that minimizes recovery time and gets students back to active status. On top of all this, somatics is fun and intriguing (What martial arts student doesn't want to feel more empowered more about his or her own body?), and therefore easily marketable.

Finally, somatics is the best way I know of for teachers to take care of themselves. Between meeting the needs of students and attending to the executive demands of managing our businesses, teachers often put ourselves last, the consequence being that we can be as prone to the long-term effects of stress and injury as anyone else. Prior to learning somatics I regularly sought out chiropractic care and deep tissue massage. I regarded those therapeutic services as just one of the costs of my doing business as I got older. Since I began my training at somatics I no longer feel the same need for massage, and my chiropractic visits have become a biannual formality instead of a biweekly necessity. A few minutes of somatic movement patterns each day are all I need now to keep my body de-stressed and free of chronic muscle tightness.

Somatics is the best overall investment any martial artist (teacher or student) can make toward extending their active participation in the arts. Well past my mid-fifties, I don't do everything just as I did when I was thirty. Yet, I don't feel that my body is in decline as such. In fact, there are things I'm able to do with my body now that were beyond my ability when I was younger. My body is smarter now. Especially, as an internal martial artist specializing in Tai Chi, I sense that my body is more aware and responsive, proprioceptively, as compared to when I was first starting out. Without those nagging and debilitating issues with lower back pain and sore joints, I feel an easy confidence about what my future portends. I feel exactly the sense of ease and comfort one ought to feel in response to any significant investment.

As a martial arts professional, I can assert that somatic education is a uniquely effective resource for managing my own health, as well as a truly effective means of contributing meaningfully to the health and well-being of those I guide. I recommend somatics for anyone committed to a pursuit of internal or external martial arts.

Distinguishing Between Somatics and Massage

In Chapter 8, I stipulated that all credible therapies can prove helpful under the right circumstances. Every therapy can work effectively for any given client, providing that therapy is exactly what that client needs at that time. Because somatics is a "body centered" modality—albeit one that is educational versus therapeutic—in which clients receive their individual sessions on massage-type tables, HSE can easily be mistaken for being one more amongst a rather broad field of massage-type therapies. Such misunderstandings can contribute to false expectations from clients.

Somatics—by which I mean both its principles and theory and also its applied practice—is sufficiently comprehensive that it will meet (at least some of) the needs of almost any person. Everybody suffers to some degree from the insults that inevitably occur over the course of a life lived. Furthermore, because of its truly unique approach, the particular needs that somatics meets in any individual person are unlikely to be addressed comprehensively by other modalities. I regard myself as a proponent of massage and other therapies when indicated; but if a client's problems are stemming from sensorimotor amnesia, any therapeutic approach that fails to address the client's problems from the perspective of SMA as the underlying cause will prove palliative at best. Body problems that are perpetuated by faulty wiring in the brain can only be set right by correcting the underlying problem at its source.

Over recent decades, massage in its many legitimate variations has proliferated, achieving a long overdue mainstream acceptance. In light of this, if you are already familiar with massage, you can anticipate that the experience of somatics table work will differ from massage in several important and defining regards. Most obviously, one of the widely touted effects of massage—in fact, the feature about massage that many people find most appealing—is that massage can be so relaxing as clients find themselves soothed into a deeply parasympathetic state. The various practice techniques of massage aside, the orchestration of this relaxation can be seen in the ambiance of many massage environments: soothing music, subdued lighting, candles, aromatics, and the like. Massage clients are encouraged to view their experience as a vacation from the trials and tribulations of daily living. In essence, clients are lulled into a subcortical state of mind and body.

Because massage is regarded as a "therapeutic" modality, the very essence of a client's experience is that a massage is being done to them, or performed on them. There is typically little, if any, emphasis on massage as an experience in which provider and client actively collaborate on the technical features of the massage in progress. In both these regards, this is exactly the opposite of the somatics experience.

Somatic education entails a highly corticalized experience in which the client plays an indispensable participatory role. The purpose of HSE is to eliminate sensorimotor amnesia and its effects. This is accomplished by helping clients to learn how to pay attention to themselves in a profoundly mindful manner, to recover full voluntary control of motor function via differentiation skills. Such applied attention requires that clients be actively intentive rather than passively receptive. As only clients themselves can exercise precise cortical awareness of their own bodies, they are at least as responsible for the ultimate results of their somatics experience as their chosen provider.

For clients who are accustomed to a therapeutic approach that works at them or on them, the HSE educational experience will certainly represent something of a departure. However, the potential benefits of self-directed care and maintenance over the long-term become rather quickly self-evident to many who opt for the HSE method.

Somatic Education as Political Commentary

This heading may seem at first a bit absurd, if not provocative. Almost everything in this book has been about getting your body to work in the best way possible. What's that got to do with politics? In its simplest guise, politics is nothing more than an expression of prevailing moral values. When we choose to move slowly and conscientiously with our bodies, we are also setting the stage for a powerful moral transformation. Many people live their lives largely on automatic pilot, which I argue creates an unlikely circumstance for conducing the first-person oversight requisite to a highly evolved morality. Automaticity is made all the more insidious because it is the social norm, and reinforced by the similar behavior of like-minded others, making for a different kind of "SMA," a social moral amnesia, if you will. Because it is "normal," just as with sensorimotor amnesia, we may hardly notice how the effects of automatic momentum, whether it be physical or mental, erode our capacity for individuality and free will.

You may recall that I cited Thomas Hanna, early on, as having been driven in his passion for helping mankind to become free. An inescapable aspect of one's being free is a sense of individuality; that is having a tenor of separateness (not to be confused with separation) from others. Inherent in this sense of separate existence lies one's ability to view oneself as truly unique, and to chart out a course of self-determination.

Over recent decades, it seems the trend here in the West has been away from separateness and individuation. Even in America, the "me" country, we retain but an illusory vestige of true individuality. Everywhere we are taught and encouraged to blend in, to conform, to go along to get along, to tow the line. The collective indoctrination starts early as young children are groomed through standardized academics (which often emphasize test scores and rote learning over critical and creative thinking), in preparation for an ever-narrowing selection of genuinely productive career choices. Insidiously, our rights as American citizens and as human beings have been subverted in such a manner that few people are even aware of our collective disempowerment. This can be seen on many levels in society, and can certainly be seen in our healthcare system—just one among many systems that is increasingly both less human and less humane—and characterized by anonymity in the name of efficiency, packaged and sold to you as being for your own ultimate good. I am troubled by this.

I believe the reason people are so sadly out of touch with their own health and well-being (the main premise of this book being people's out-of-touchness with their own bodies and what to do about it) is as much a reflection on the body politic and its propensity for social moral amnesia as it is commentary at the level of the individual. This notwithstanding, it remains for each of us our own responsibility to initiate change, at least at our own individual level, in what amounts to a more deeply personal application of the adage, "Think globally, act locally." Not everyone can change geopolitical patterns or government corruption, apathy, or special interests. But we can each empower ourselves in a way that makes a difference in how we experience living in our own bodies.

Somatics bucks the disenfranchisement trend. The movement patterns and pandiculations of somatics are good for you for all the many reasons enumerated throughout this book. In addition, your ability to experience your body in a differentiated fashion provides a model for differentiating your very self to accomplish a true autonomy. Arguably, the essence of Thomas Hanna's somatics is to foment sedition against the body politic's complacent and automatic ethic at a deep personal level to accomplish the most free, the most self-determined, and most evolved you. By learning how to individuate muscular functions and motor behaviors, you are, in a real and practical way, asserting your capacity for individuality and separateness, and for personal freedom and a more evolved personal morality. Where better to start taking charge of yourself than in your own body? Individuation is something that nobody can do to you or for you, but something only you can do for yourself. In learning to assert your own individuality you can become free according to the most essential meaning of the concept.

CHAPTER 11

NEUROPHYSIOLOGICAL PERSPECTIVES

Distinguishing Between SMA and Its Causes and Effects

There is no doubt that somatic education can effectively redress neuromuscular pain and stiffness, which is to say, *it really works*. However, as is the case with homeopathic remedies (many of which have been in use, unchanged, since the 1700s), and also like a number of more conventional pharmaceutical drugs that have been employed "off label" because they are known empirically to work despite not having been subjected to current drug testing standards,[1] a scientifically precise and fully detailed understanding of exactly how somatics works lags somewhat behind its known efficacy. We have a detailed grasp of the neurophysiological causes and effects involved, but we do not have *all* the answers. I do not mean to suggest that somatics is based on weak science, or that HSE has a weak basis in good science. On the contrary, somatics is solidly founded in conventional neurophysiology. I mean only to explain that, like any of the other relatively recent applications in the rapidly developing brain/body field, an exact and fully comprehensive explanation of the specific neurophysiological mechanisms underlying SMA (and its orchestrated redress by qualified somatic educators) continues to reveal itself commensurate with ongoing advances in the neurosciences. In other words, we're a developing field, just like many of the other fields with a basis in neuroscience; and just like these other fields, or even entirely separate fields like mathematics or astrophysics, new developments will continue to shed fresh light on the understandings we already have about our particular area of

---

1 Examples of untested drugs include aspirin and acetaminophen. Others drugs may be used off label for conditions for which they've not been tested, e.g., amitryptiline for IBS, diazepam for hypertension.

expertise and why it works as effectively as it does. What we do know beyond a shadow of a doubt is that somatics is effective in a large number of cases at resolving neuromuscular pain and postural dissonance.

Though sensorimotor amnesia is a de facto reality of life for many people saddled with its burdensome limitations, the concept of SMA as such, and its labeling as *the* identifiable cause of those limitations, remains more or less exclusive to the realm of educators trained in the tradition of Thomas Hanna. This is true to the extent that Thomas Hanna was the first person to recognize sensorimotor amnesia for what it is, and label it as such. Hanna pioneered the concept that chronic muscular engagement is rooted in faulty patterns imprinted on the neural circuitry. He then went on to fashion a bone fide educational/ preventative/ restorative healthcare system around his brainchild.

As an aside, one might wonder that for all the seeming potential of the human brain, it makes little sense that the brain would even allow, let alone abet, a process such as sensorimotor amnesia. After all, isn't it the brain's role to protect the integrity of the organism that houses it? How is it that the human brain did not evolve with internal self-adjusting mechanisms to correct problems such as SMA? These days even our cars tell us when they need preventative maintenance or corrective service. Surely, the brain must be more advanced in this regard than the family car. The answer may lie in how the brain evolved.

Rather than having developed into its current form from an original master blueprint designed to cover all contingencies, such as occurs when a skilled architect designs elaborate plans prior to the construction of a skyscraper, the evolution of the human brain is more akin to a rambling New England farmhouse onto which various additions have been added as the need arose, leaving us with what is regarded by some as the tripartite brain.[2]

---

2   The concept of a *tripartite brain* distinguishes between the brainstem, the limbic system, and the cerebral cortex as separate components of the brain. Accordingly, these three components evolved over time as the need arose. They are understood to develop and mature in any given individual sequentially rather than simultaneously, leaving each of these brain divisions with separate and distinct, though usually well-integrated, roles in the mature body.

Consequently, advanced as they may appear, the processing systems of the brain are not always seamless. The mailroom and the executive offices don't always see eye to eye in operating according to the same agenda. Sensorimotor amnesia may be, for all we know at this time, the result of the brain's best effort to cope in organizing and managing the body as best it can, given the limits of its design.

What then is sensorimotor amnesia, and what is it not? Sensorimotor amnesia, by definition (albeit simplistic), is a kind of "forgetting," characterized by the brain's having become compromised in its ability to fully control and differentiate the function and performance of certain voluntary muscles. Somewhat less simplistically, alpha motor neurons innervate extrafusal muscle fiber. Their role is to contract voluntary muscle, and also to maintain a steady resting tonus in the muscles, tonus being understood as the amount of continuous force exerted by a muscle while in a relaxed, or passive, state sufficient to oppose stretching. Meanwhile, gamma motor neurons innervate intrafusal muscle fiber. Their role is to regulate the sensitivity of the muscle spindles—to establish the baseline tonus for the extrafusal fibers—so that as the intrafusal muscle fibers contract only a small stretch is required to activate spindle sensory neurons and also the stretch reflex as a protective mechanism. The upshot is that alpha and gamma motor neurons must work collaboratively in a coactive fashion for there to be optimal muscle function. Such coactivation can become compromised for any number of reasons, such as blatant disease processes, or from the various kinds of insults as already discussed.

Vernon B. Brooks, author of *The Neural Basis of Motor Control,* opined that Hanna's method of assisted pandiculation effectively resets the coactivation of alpha-gamma motor neurons (AG-MN).[3] Deconstructing Brooks' statement suggests that sensorimotor amnesia, therefore, has something to do with (and perhaps even results from) alpha-gamma motor neurons *not* coactivating in a correct manner. This leaves me wondering if SMA might be,

---

3 This reportedly occurred when a gathering of Hanna somatic educators hosted Brooks for a guest appearance some years ago, as per personal correspondence.

at least to some extent, explained by a corollary of Hebb's Law,[4] the corollary being that "neurons that don't fire together, don't wire together." When the firing of alpha-gamma motor neurons is not properly coactivated, the brain no longer receives fully accurate information on the status of the muscle fibers those neurons innervate. Absenting that information, the brain loses its basis for voluntary motor control of those fibers. Without oversight by the brain, muscles normally do one of three things: 1) muscles can contract and the contraction can be maintained as chronic hypertonus (the most common cause of this being SMA), 2) muscles can relax and remain flaccid and limp (hypotonic), or 3) muscles can vacillate between the two former states. The latter two responses generally stem from debilitating or traumatic neurological conditions or events. In the former case, when the loss of neural oversight is due to the aforementioned alpha-gamma motor neuron non-coactivation factor, your brain is deprived of pertinent information. This serves as a basis for adopting an errant, hypertonic, default pattern for the muscle(s) or muscle fibers (or more properly, motor units) in question.

The questions I ponder here are these: Are sensorimotor amnesia, on the one hand, and its underlying causes, along with the muscular habituation that ensues, on the other hand, all one and same issue? Or, are they different but intertwined facets of a more comprehensive issue? If they are intertwined, are they unintertwinable—that is, can the causes of SMA, the neural manifestation of SMA, and the effects of SMA (as habituated patterns in muscle tissue occurring away from the brain) exist as separate from each other? Can one have patterns of habituation without SMA? Or, can one have SMA without patterns of habituation? And, if these various concerns can exist as separate, however intertwined, entities what light might that shed on the best way to undo whatever damaging or limiting effects they may impose? I don't have the answers to all these questions, but posing the questions makes for some interesting reflection. Let's start with a closer look at the causes of sensorimotor amnesia.

---

4   Canadian psychologist, Donald Hebb, introduced the concept, circa 1940s, that "neurons that fire together wire together."

Sensorimotor amnesia is caused or initiated by some manner of insult to a muscle. The initiating insult can stem from a blatant direct cause such as traumatic injury, i.e. a blow, or from overuse issues such as submitting the body to ergonomically incorrect stressors beyond its ability to self-correct, or even indirectly from emotional stressors or other causes. Notably, not every insult results in SMA. Some insults are sufficiently benign that they fail to evoke an apparent SMA response. Other, less mild, insults may still fall within a range of the body's ability to self-correct. The lodging of insults, as well as the totality of their impact, can also vary according to the resilience of the individual and according to any predispositions stemming from the effects of previous insults.

However, once the insult or insults have reached a certain critical threshold that surpasses the body's self-correcting abilities—enough so that there ensues a communication breakdown between muscle and brain[5]—it seems that the brain habituates itself to the body's reaction to the insult. Curiously, this can happen over time and incrementally in response to repeated low-level insults, or almost instantaneously in response to blatant trauma. Exactly how this happens depends to a large extent on the resilience or susceptibility of any given individual. Once that threshold has been passed the brain responds by adopting a new and errant default pattern for that muscle.[6] The new, errant, default state always entails some degree of chronic muscular contraction, whether it be an almost unnoticeable fraction of a percent up to a significant degree of hypertonus (an extreme example of hypertonus being tetanus) sufficient to cause pain or obvious postural distortion.

Let me hasten to add that not every occurrence of habituation is pathological. Habituation describes any behavior that is determined by force of habit. Clearly, some habits can be benign, such as if you are asked to interlace the fingers of your hands quickly and without forethought. Absenting your

---

5   References herein to the brain are inclusive of the CNS.
6   A default setting establishes a muscle's baseline tonus when it is not being deliberately recruited for an action.

conscious intention to perform otherwise, you will invariably interlace your hands in the same manner each and every time. You're just as likely to step without forethought each time you dress into your trousers with the same leg first. These are habits, yes, but not ones for which I assess any pathological effect. What difference, after all, does it make how you interlace your fingers or put on your pants? Habituation only becomes problematic when it causes problems, such as typically ensue from the *archeology of insults* introduced in Chapter 1 (though, hypothetically, even interlacing your fingers in a habituated manner could be problematic if you needed to operate outside the pattern, e.g., if you were a professional finger interlacer).

Now, let's look more closely at the effects, as they occur in your body, of habituation in your brain. Muscular habituation is what happens when a muscle adopts a behavior other than its normal or relaxed state (meaning any state of abnormal contraction) as its default mode. One effect stemming from the habit of a muscle held in inadvertent contraction[7] is to interfere with the efficiency of afferent nerve impulses, whose duty it is to report on that muscle's status or performance to the brain. This interference, in turn, hinders the brain's ability to sense and control the muscle. In this manner, habituated behaviors, by themselves, are a primary cause of sensorimotor amnesia,[8] not the other way around. Therefore, de-habituation is one effective means of facilitating *sensorimotor recollection*, or *SMR*, if you will. In HSE we facilitate de-habituation by resetting the coactivation of alpha-gamma motor neurons through assisted and self-pandiculation techniques. Resetting the coactivation of motor neurons in the targeted muscle allows its "neurons to fire together in order to wire together," ala Hebb, so that accurate sensory information from the muscles can serve as a basis for the brain in exercising intelligent and informed motor command.

Rest easy here, though. As a somatics client it won't be necessary to grasp

---

7   The word "inadvertent" makes for an important distinction as the default tonus for striated muscles can be variable, e.g., the pteragoid muscles, and some sphincter and perineal muscles have higher resting tonus.

8   This is usually true, except when some other factor is at cause, e.g., stroke.

all the technical terms and theory behind this to enjoy full benefit.

As noted, not all habituation is bad. A force of habit is, after all, nothing more than that which the brain has accustomed itself to, or prioritized as a memory, and which has been relegated to implicit memory or function.

Even though it is usually muscle dysfunction that causes sensorimotor amnesia in the brain, it is in the brain, and not just at the location of the expression of a problem in the muscles, where corrective measures must be implemented. Once muscles have entered into an habituated state the pattern becomes imprinted in the brain, specifically in the subcortex.[9] Imprints can be so thoroughly encoded into the brain as to supersede their underlying causes, even to a point of surviving the causative muscular habituation. Such surviving imprints can often be seen in cases of phantom pain in missing limbs.[10] This resistance to imprint extinction is exactly why individuals seeking relief from muscle tension or discomfort via massage-type modalities often feel better initially, only to have their problems recur as the errant pattern reasserts itself. If the problem itself can outlive the underlying cause, we must consider this as evidence that the underlying cause and the problem itself are not one and the same.

Neuroscientist V.S. Ramachandran described working with amputee patients regarding their experiences of phantom limbs, citing cases in which patients were reportedly aware of pronounced somatic dispositions in their missing parts. In the described cases, patients reported experiencing discomfort, spasms, or outright agony in physically nonexistent limbs as if those limbs were present. These reports provide compelling testimony that errant brain patterns can survive the habituations that caused them. Ramachandran reported inducing in his research subjects the "perception" of voluntary control of the missing limb, which allowed him to introduce methods to ame-

---

9 Thomas Hanna, *Somatics. Healing Arts Press,* 1988.

10 See V.S. Ramachandran, *Phantoms In the Brain,* Quill, 1998, pp. 43-46, for a discussion of how paralysis can be "learned" by a body part due to preexisting pathology, only to become imprinted into the brain's circuitry in a manner that survives subsequent loss or removal of that body part.

liorate the patients' discomfort or pain.[11] His method for accomplishing this is both fascinating and brilliant, not to mention refreshingly low tech, but secondary in its importance to the point being made here—that the changes he induced to manage pain and discomfort in missing limbs occurred entirely in the brain, not in the limb itself. To implement lasting amelioration in cases of muscular habituation the primary focal point for change needs to be in the brain, not in the muscles.

Let's return to my earlier assertion that habituated patterns cause sensorimotor amnesia, versus the other way around. Consider the following experiment as a way you could put this to the test [do NOT try this]. If you were to deliberately engage in an activity that causes insult—for example a repetitive or long-lasting activity in an ergonomically incorrect posture (something I do every time I sit down at my computer to write for hours on end)—you could push beyond mere fatigue to induce habituated muscle tonus, for which sensorimotor amnesia might well ensue. However, if you tried to accomplish the reverse [this you can try]—for example, to think about a muscle behavior for which you want to deliberately induce SMA, only *without first* causing habituation—you not only could not do that, but you would accomplish just the exact opposite. Instead of your brain forgetting about that muscle, you would develop a heightened awareness of the very thing you were trying to forget. If you tell somebody to not think about the big toe on their right foot, it will immediately, even if just momentarily, command that person's attention.

Naturally, there are an infinite number of awarenesses about your body that your brain could have, but does not have, at any given time. For the most part, these are not lapses in your brain, and they certainly are not tantamount to sensorimotor amnesia. You could decide at any time to focus your attention on a particular body part to assert your voluntary control over it. The setting of attentional priorities is nature's way of protecting you from sensory overload through the brain's natural filtering mechanisms. The upshot is that you could use your mind, electively, to induce muscular habituation to cause

---

11 Ramachandran, *A Brief Tour*.

SMA, but not induce sensorimotor amnesia to cause muscular habituation.

Sensorimotor amnesia is, thus, both the result of habituated muscle patterns, as I've illustrated above, and its unwitting partner. Beyond its being the result of chronic muscular engagement, sensorimotor amnesia does, however, serve to reinforce the very problem that caused it. Any errant patterns of habituation existing in the body have no ability, or reason, to change on their own—to be anything other than habituated, which is to say stuck—for the duration of the brain's "amnesia" to them. If (and once) the brain is able to resume full awareness of the forgotten muscle function, it will thereby have the means to undo the habit, but not before. An important point to keep in mind is that the brain can only control voluntary muscles voluntarily to whatever extent it has a conscious awareness of those muscles. The brain can't control voluntarily what it can't sense. From this, we can see that sensorimotor amnesia and habituation are not one and the same, however intertwined they may be, despite that these terms are casually invoked interchangeably. Rather, one stems from the other, leading them to become mutually reinforcing dynamics.

Given this relationship, how likely or possible is it that sensorimotor amnesia and the effects of the insults that lead to it might exist as separate from each other? In other words, what happens if we try to "fix the problem" by addressing it only in the muscle (where SMA is experienced as problematic) while the errant default pattern in the brain remains intact? This is already a common scenario, as therapeutic modalities such as massage or physical therapy, and a host of others, typically do just that. If, perchance, the quality of massage is high, and the extent of damage or limitation to the muscle is minimal and short-standing so that a new and errant default pattern has not become firmly established (a problem, yes, but actual SMA, no), then massage may provide local relief along with an opportunity for the body's natural healing mechanisms to take over. From what I've seen, however, the more widespread or longstanding an issue, or especially if there are preexisting complications also involving SMA, the smaller the likelihood that the initial benefits stemming from massage (or any therapeutic modality) will endure.

More often, the underlying problems are simply palliated, or deferred. What we then end up with is a revolving-door syndrome as clients feel initially better following treatment, only to relapse after a short while, or remain prone to relapse. That muscular problems may be rooted in errant default patterns in the brain goes a long way in explaining why clients of providers whose therapeutic methods fail to take this into account often need to seek out treatment on a regular and ongoing basis for the same recurring problems. This makes for the revolving door.

Suppose we reverse this scenario. Suppose we try to repair the problem in the muscle by merely thinking about changing the pattern in the brain, say, by "meditating" on it without deliberately synchronizing engagement of the muscle in question. Hypothetically, that's possible, given the power the brain wields as evidenced by Ramachandra's research on phantom limbs and Paul Bach-y-Rita's research on motor learning. Keep in mind though that in orchestrating a new neural default pattern, Ramachandran substituted the actual muscular engagement of a real (opposite) limb as an imaginary replacement for one that was missing. Also, Bach-y-Rita's orchestrated activation of motor neurons, accomplished by having subjects imagine a motor action, is still a ways from releasing long-held muscular tensions. Though I wouldn't discount this approach as altogether impossible under ideal conditions, it would seem to require a level of self-sensing quite beyond the skills of most people. Tangible results in recalibrating errant patterns in the brain are still most likely to be accomplished through a synchronized engagement of problem muscles and neural oversight. In order to produce effective and lasting change in muscles that suffer from chronic engagement and pain, we must coordinate direct attention to the muscles with the purposeful (cortical) intention of the mind. A fully integrated mind/body approach is likely to produce the best results.

It's time now to turn our attention to how we can make the benefits of HSE a habit onto themselves. Remember, not all habituations are bad for us. We just need to consider adding a new, desirable habit to our repertoire of personal behaviors. Part of learning *about* somatics includes how to make the best use of what we've learned.

To gain lasting benefit from any somatics movement patterns you learn, you must integrate them into your daily routine. This sounds simple, but for many people the habituation of their daily lives that got them into trouble initially will prevent them from prioritizing personal maintenance work. Some people are just disinclined to keep up their home practice patterns and continually reinforce the gains they have made. This can even include folks who have already obtained good results from their clinical sessions or home movement practices, but then discontinued or neglected their practice, leaving themselves unknowingly susceptible to relapse. This begs the question—how do you make your personal somatics practice a top priority? Prioritization boils down to values. The setting of priorities hinges on your own personal values. People prioritize those behaviors that reflect the values they hold.

Imagine this strange scenario: there is an advanced culture of individuals who are well educated and perfectly capable of thinking critically to assume full responsibility for their own health and well-being. However, instead of choosing to live in the healthiest manner possible, these individuals are accustomed to smoking, overindulging in alcohol, or eating unhealthy food in excess such that obesity becomes rampant. They eschew healthy exercise habits in favor of mindless pursuits like watching TV for hours on end. They cease formal education beyond high school or college age, and subsequently fail to take initiative in making intelligent, proactive, and well-informed decisions about their own healthcare. Unbelievably, the people of this culture choose, instead, to allow the most important decisions determining their own quality of life to be made for them by other, purportedly knowledgeable, authority figures, often without question. Sound familiar? Now ask yourself, does that sound sensible? Not very. Yet this is an apt description of modern life, and of how many individuals live. Careful reflection regarding personal priorities may influence you to readjust the values you place on your health and well-being, to scrutinize and adjust your personal values, and reassign your health the priority it deserves so that you can live your life to the fullest. Nobody else can do that for you. You must do this for yourself, and your future starts now.

Various Types of Habituation

It might surprise you to reflect on some other areas where we can all be prone to habituation. The effects of pathological habituation, such as we address in somatics, are physiologic. They occur in the muscles. However, habituation is not confined to muscles. Habituation (and here I use this term loosely) can manifest in mental/cognitive processes, in the emotional realm, and with other forms of sensory functions or expressions, e.g., the quality of one's voice or facial expressions. There may even be some extent to which dermal appearances have some basis in habituation. Let's take a closer look at these.

Mental (Emotional or Cognitive) Habituation

One expression of mental habituation may be seen in a stubborn or "closed" mind, or a mind that is prone to linear and non-creative thinking, or in conditions such as OCD (obsessive compulsive disorder). Dr. Jeffery M. Schwartz discussed what he calls "brain lock" in his pioneering work with OCD patients.[12] His approach focuses on dehabituating certain brain functions by repatterning the neural intransigence of those suffering from this disorder to counter the effects of brain lock. Less clinically, a closed mind is one that has splinted itself, or dissociated, against thoughts, beliefs, or realities that may challenge the validity of whatever thoughts or beliefs it already holds. A closed mind may *not want* to change and has limited tolerance for anything that challenges its status quo. Mental habituation can be seen in political or religious zealotry, in "isms," e.g., racism, sexism, communism, terrorism, jingoism, etc., often involving bigotry or intolerance. According to Schwartz,

---

12 Jeffery M. Schwartz, M.D. and Sharon Begley argue convincingly for a neural basis for such conditions as OCD in their book, *The Mind and the Brain: Neuroplasticity and the Power of Mental Force*, ReganBooks, 2002.

brain lock issues have a self-reinforcing basis in neural programming. This sentiment was echoed by Louis Cozolino Ph.D. when he asserted, "...belief perseverance is our tendency to attend to facts that support our beliefs while we ignore those that contradict our beliefs." Cozolino added, "Belief perseverance is the enemy of neural plasticity."[13] This is important because bodies and minds can both reflect and reinforce each other's *tendency* for stuckness. An intransigent mind can predispose one to a stuck body.

Emotional/cognitive habituation can also be seen as various phobias or neuroses; though it's important to note there may be more to such conditions than just simply habituation.[14] Other, less overtly pathological, emotional issues such as rational anger, sadness, or grief that have been retained despite having outlived their rational usefulness, can also represent examples of habituated emotions. Powerful emotions often take on a life of their own, generated by their own momentum. You probably know people whose propensity for sadness, anger, or emotional imbalance defines them. Cozolino described how traumatic emotional responses can result even from non-life-threatening experiences, such as tension-packed households, peer pressure, or chronic loneliness. It makes sense to imagine how such emotionally based trauma might express itself neuromuscularly, as people adopt unconscious armatures in response to their environments or perceived experiences.

A whole other category of psychologically based muscular habituation can be seen in (some) cases of conversion disorder, a psychological condition so called because it is believed emotional anxiety becomes somehow converted into physical symptoms. In such circumstances persons can display seemingly neurological-based symptoms, e.g., muscular paralysis, for which no neurological basis can be assessed.

---

13   Cozolino, *The Neuroscience*.
14   To suggest that emotional pathologies are nothing more than habituation would be an irresponsible oversimplification. Hormones, biochemicals, and neurotransmitters can all affect both mental and emotional states and behaviors. Yet, phobias or neuroses often involve some element of an ingrained pattern contributing to the expression of the condition.

Teleceptor Habituation

The brain can also habituate as per teleceptors—sight or hearing or smell—accustoming to certain select stimuli, aka apperceptive attention,[15] to the exclusion of others. If you're a city dweller who has ever spent a night camping in the woods, the quiet at night may have kept you awake. Or, if you hail from quieter quarters, trying to sleep through your first night of city screechings, blarings, and general urban cacophony can take some getting used to. Every mother knows how attuned her hearing becomes for the sounds of a newborn infant, even while other more pronounced noises may be filtered out. Ironically, it will be that same infant who, fifteen years hence as a teenager, habitually filters out his parents' remonstrations.

Teleceptor senses, like any others, tend to habituate according to the familiarity and perceived significance of their experiences. Of course, with teleceptors the brain has a self-adjusting plasticity. Given time and incentive, the brain is able to reinterpret external data as it adjusts to new priorities and stimuli, which is to say it can learn. Other, non-sensory apparatus such as one's voice, though not a teleceptor, can also reflect factors that have caused it to become habituated. That habituations in the body can undermine the quality of one's voice is no small consideration for actors, singers, and orators. An early pioneer in the somatic field was F. Matthias Alexander, the Australian stage actor who developed his Alexander Technique, a predecessor of modern somatics.

Other Effects of Habituation

Even such unlikely aspects as one's dermal surface may reflect underlying habituations. Think of facial wrinkles that may be caused or exacerbated by chronic stress levels. Each of us has more than one hundred individual muscles

---

15 James, *The Principles.*

involved in movements of our head, neck, face, jaw, and eyes alone.[16] Unlike the majority of striated (motor) muscles located elsewhere in the body that attach via tendons from bone to bone, many of these facial muscles attach directly to the skin. Your facial skin is quite sensitive to even small stresses in the underlying musculature. If people could learn how to ease their stress levels and relax the muscles of their face, they might eliminate the "need" for Botox and many of the other purported remedies pandered to mask or undo the appearances of aging.

Not All Habituation is Bad

The fact is that individuals can become habituated to just about anything the brain filters out, as well as to the same stimuli the brain prioritizes. Habituation is simply a euphemism for that which the brain has accustomed itself to as normal and standard, its status quo so to speak. In some cases habituation even confers certain advantages. William James noted, "Habit simplifies the movements required to achieve given result, makes them more accurate and diminishes fatigue...habit diminishes the conscious attention with which our acts are performed."[17] James did caution, however, "Keep the faculty of effort alive in you by a little gratuitous exercise every day. That is, be systematically ascetic or heroic in little unnecessary points, do every day or two something for no other reason than that you would rather not do it, so that when the hour of dire need draws nigh, it may find you not unnerved and untrained to stand the test."

Again, habituation is not inherently bad. There is nothing even remotely unhealthy about being in the habit of waking up every morning at sunrise (though late risers may beg to differ). Some forms of habituation are the brain's way of insuring that we function safely and effectively in our normal predictable environment.

---

16 Daniel Goleman, *Social Intelligence*, Bantom, 2006, cites Paul Ekman Ph.D., an expert in the field, as noting nearly 200 such muscles, p. 44.
17 James, *The Principles*.

Habituation does, however, become problematic when it is characterized by stuckness, or the inability to operate electively in an unhabituated manner given the need to do so.

The human organism is characterized by its ability to adapt advantageously to wide-ranging change. Loss or reduction of one's ability to adapt forespeaks a trajectory of decline. Collectively, such loss represents an evolutionary regression of the species. This, I fear, makes for one possible future scenario as people increasingly lose the ability to find genuine touch with themselves.

What then determines whether or not the effects of some real or perceived experience become habituated as patterns of stuckness in your body or mind? More to the point, how can these unhealthy patterns of stuckness be dispensed with? In cases of unconscious mutually reinforcing dynamics, such as when you have both sensorimotor amnesia and its effects in muscular habituation, your best bet in managing or eliminating them may start with simply bringing them (or having them brought) to the conscious fore. This is exactly the approach we take in somatics, by asking clients to consciously and purposefully attend to aspects of their bodies that have been forgotten, so that differentiation and voluntary muscular control can be effectively restored.

Taijiquan and Somatics

I am enamored of a marriage close to my heart. Taijiquan and somatic education make for perfect bedfellows, having direct and immediate relevance to each other in their mutually supporting dynamics. In both cases, expertise (at Tai Chi) and efficacy (at somatics) can be enhanced in no small measure by the influence of the other.

In Tai Chi, expertise is gauged in one's ability to differentiate, at a subtle level, the structural articulations and muscular nuances necessary to manage effort and transfer force through the physical body with optimal efficiency, all while *rooting* to the earth and maintaining an easy sense of equilibrium and congruence overall. Achieving these goals can prove problematic for persons saddled with sensorimotor amnesia as SMA precludes the requisite sensitivity for *listening* to and controlling one's body in an appropriately precise fashion. Somatics is a perfect companion practice for students of Tai Chi as mastery at Tai Chi hinges on "knowing your body" and being able to exercise full voluntary control over your motor system. Somatics can shave years, perhaps decades, from the time otherwise required to reach a level of personal competence, or mastery at Tai Chi. Somatics can eliminate impediments to skillful Tai Chi and afford you a smarter body in the process.

This relationship between HSE and Tai Chi is reciprocal, though; as Tai Chi can also enhance one's experience of somatics. With somatics, efficacy is measured in the ease and freedom with which one is able to experience and manage one's body. Somatics is wonderfully effective at undoing the causes of sensorimotor amnesia to restore neuromuscular freedom and control. However, one of the very features that renders somatics so effective is that its patterns are (generally) practiced in a lying down position; this allows the body to differentiate outside the usual constraints of gravity.

This same feature, however, may also serve to challenge its practical application once an activity is resumed in an upright posture. Having grasped the subtler benefits of somatics in a lying or sitting posture, these benefits may not translate quite automatically while standing or walking about in one's usual manner. Tai Chi offers the prospect of reinforcing those benefits commensurate with the somatics model of proprioceptive self-sensing. Tai Chi accomplishes this by engaging the body directly and very deliberately with the same gravitational forces that might otherwise invite and reinforce relapse into old errant patterns. Furthermore, Tai Chi offers the prospect of expanded practical application of newfound HSE-derived abilities. It provides an effective model for moving with enhanced sensorial awareness while navigating your body seamlessly through the process of daily living.

When I practice Tai Chi, I am continually aware of the influence of somatics on my overall Tai Chi experience. Conversely, when I engage in practice at somatics, either on my own for myself or as a provider in collaboration with clients on my table, I am ever sensitive to the nuances and listening skills afforded me by the Tai Chi model. Each of these disciplines seems to foster a receptivity for the other, rendering them as compatible and mutually reinforcing—even necessary to each other—as are two sides of a same coin. Anyone who is committed to a practice and study of one should consider undertaking some study, at the least, of the other.

Somatics, Tai Chi, and Your Brain

As noted, competence at Tai Chi hinges on knowing your body and having a highly refined ability to self-sense for full voluntary control. There are many ways that one can develop self-sensing skills. I've noted here two methods for improving proprioception and voluntary muscular control as required for Taijiquan.

The first method is the easier and more natural of the two, and is probably what you already do, albeit unconsciously, if you are an experienced Tai Chi practitioner. This method entails making your best effort at noticing, at being consciously mindful, of whatever your body is doing. Wait a minute, did I just contradict myself? Which is it? Are we being conscious or unconscious? To be clear, you are being conscious about your Tai Chi, but quite probably unconscious about being conscious about your Tai Chi. Most Tai Chi players learn to pay close attention to *what* they're practicing. However, paying attention on an even deeper level than "what" entails yet another level of development.

In Taijiquan, your sensorial awareness is already heightened by the fact that you move slowly, so that the movement, or doing, itself serves as a primary focal point. This heightened awareness of doing represents an improvement for most people in any case as people typically go along through their lives according to an unconscious momentum, running on automatic pilot as it were. Experiencing some degree of deeper-than-usual awareness of one's self while engaged at Tai Chi is quite natural as the brain is wired to observe the most commanding stimulus dished up before it. This is especially so if the stimulus occurs in the first person—if your own body is doing the dishing—and slowly at that. Whatever your body may be doing already primes the brain for a certain quality of attention. The slowness of Tai Chi focuses and amplifies the brain's attention, given the brain's natural affinity for novelty. Yet, there's a limit to whatever extent the mere act of moving slowly can hold the brain's attention. Sooner or later even the slowness of Tai Chi will exhaust its novelty factor.

This is where the second method comes into play. This second method involves performing an action or behavior, e.g. Tai Chi, but "according to your brain's intention to notice 'what' happens, as well as 'how' and 'why'" at a subtler level. The difference between these two approaches is that in the first case your brain is only observing whatever may already be happening. In the second case your brain is also participating in the action, so that your experience of observing your Tai Chi becomes, itself, part of the action. In other words, you become conscious not only of the doing of Tai Chi practice, but of the process and experience of being conscious.[18]

You might liken this to the difference between a movie director who merely directs a film and one who also decides to act in the film as he is directing it. In the latter case he operates simultaneously from the dual perspective of director and actor. Here, it is not just the doing that compels your attention, but the compounded experience of paying attention to paying attention. As your agenda shifts

---

18   This is known in neuro-speak as "meta-cognition," meaning your ability to think about thinking.

and expands from focusing on the action of Tai Chi, to the underlying process of that action, you can begin to operate simultaneously from a first- and a third-person perspective. Your brain attunes to its first-person experience of self, as well as to the third-person perspective of directing and observing your body's behavior. This dual perspective entails more than merely being present to the moment immediately at hand (an oft invoked benefit of Tai Chi practice), but to the larger gestalt of that moment. Daniel Siegal described this interoception-induced phenomenon as facilitating a kind of "metamap capacity, enabling us to be one step removed from the direct sense of the body..." for an enhanced "...awareness of self."[19]

The great value in this approach is that aspects of your brain function, which might not otherwise be activated, are recruited into service. Baring this more deeply mindful approach, as Tai Chi enthusiasts practice their discipline over time, a familiarity and a possible ensuing quality of rote sets in. As familiarity sets in, the novelty of the experience diminishes, creating some risk that practice will become increasingly relegated to implicit, or automatic, memory, and with it a decrease in the real or perceived value of Tai Chi as a personal development resource. Even that part of the brain that remains cortically involved will probably allot incrementally less novelty oriented real estate over time to the task of practice, meaning there is increasingly less involvement by those parts of the brain concerned with executive functions.

However, during our second scenario, the act of paying attention to paying attention while your body is engaged at Tai Chi serves to continually excite the brain's sense of novelty. As your experience of practice transcends even the novelty of being in the moment, that moment expands to include perceived relevant realities from the past, along with anticipated relevant possibilities for the future.

---

19 Siegal, *The Mindful Therapist*.

Your Tai Chi becomes timeless and engenders an infinite capacity for additional and deeper learning by ensuring that your experience of the form remains optimally cortical and explicit, or executive, versus subcortical and implicit.

According to Siegal, this level of personal attunement promotes the three aspects of neuroplasticity: synaptogenisis, neurogenisis, and myelinogenesis. Myelinogensis, in particular, can serve to greatly enhance (on the order of three thousand times) the conduction speed of neuronal impulses.[20] Imagine that! The slower and more mindfully your move, the faster and more efficiently your brain and body become able to process information about you and your Tai Chi. As you might surmise, this makes for a substantively different and more fully encompassing Tai Chi experience than simply "going through the moves."

Absenting sophisticated measuring techniques such as fMRI to identify the specific brain areas involved, I can only speculate on which brain regions, exactly, are involved according to either method. Again, you can rest easy, as there's no need to memorize the following.

Based on the known, or suspected, roles of different brain regions, I expect this second method involves greater participation from, at least, the cerebellum (mediates and modulates proprioception with motor function), the dorsalateral prefrontal cortex (directs the focus of attention, organizes working memory, processes voluntary movements according to higher order instructions including the learning of motor sequences),[21] the medial prefrontal cortex (relates to first-person experiential awareness),[22] the basal ganglia (concerned with pattern execution),[23] the anterior insula (perceives bodily sensations),[24] the hippocampus (organizes memories of the

---

20 Ibid.
21 Cozolino, *The Neuroscience*.
22 David Rock, *Your Brain at Work*, Harper Collins, 2009.
23 Ibid.
24 Ibid.

past to form coherent mental images which may be correspondingly apropos as a basis for imagining future scenarios),[25] the left supramarginal gyrus (required for conjuring up internal images), and aspects of the limbic system (drawn into play when there is any emotional component, such as that inspired by novel experience involved with a motor task), as well as enhancing the presence of theta waves (believed to be involved in spatial learning and navigation) and gamma waves (associated with the experience of insight).[26]

Jeffery M. Schwartz M.D. referred to the brain's propensity for somatosensory "rezoning...in response to purposeful behavior."[27] He described an experiment in which subjects' brains were shown to change in response to physical stimuli, but only when the task was accompanied by the subjects' undistracted attention. Schwartz was describing experiments with monkeys, and even "purposeful" monkeys are not the same as methodical Tai Chi practitioners. Nevertheless, I am excited by the prospect suggested by Schwartz's model—that the purposefulness of the brain coupled with its focused attention to a given behavior can prioritize (even rezone) regions in the brain according to demand, presumably allotting increased neuro-resources to the task at hand. To put it in the vernacular, practicing in a deeply attentive and purposeful, or intentive, manner "keeps the shine on the apple" to insure that your practice commands your brain's fullest attention for optimal skill development. This would bode well for practitioners of Taijiquan.

This quality of self/sensorial awareness is not easily imparted to casual students of Taijiquan. Speaking as a Tai Chi teacher with four decades of teaching experience, I assure you that it can be quite challenging to impart the basics of even the former method—simply

25 Karl K. Szpunar and Kathleen B. McDermott, *Cerebrum*. Dana Press, 2008. See Chapter 2: "Remembering the Past to Imagine the Future."
26 Rock, *Your Brain*.
27 Schwartz and Begley, *The Mind*.

moving slowly enough to become more sensorially aware—let alone guiding students in the nuances of truly deep self-sensing. Just getting students to decelerate to a point where they can experience Tai Chi according to the former model can require years of tutelage. Guiding students in achieving the skills and resources requisite for the latter model might ordinarily require decades of disciplined training.

Though any Tai Chi practitioner could, theoretically, train himself or herself as described above, such achievement is highly unlikely. I practiced Tai Chi and assorted internal disciplines for nearly forty years and it wasn't until I underwent training at somatics that it occurred to me how I might apply the principles of conscious self-sensing, aka interoception via Hanna's model, to advance my Tai Chi to a deeper level. Excuse the cliché, but the effect of somatics on my Tai Chi represented a quantum leap forward for me. After I began practicing somatics on a regular basis, experiencing this deeper connection in my Tai Chi seemed like a "no-brainer." Self-sensing skills, such as these, are an integral part of the somatics experience. The acquisition of profoundly conscious self-sensing skills for Tai Chi can be streamlined with somatics as a co-practice.

CHAPTER 12

IFAQS–

INFREQUENTLY ASKED QUESTIONS

This section offers transcripts of answers (not covered elsewhere) to questions I have been asked by somatics students or clients.

Q. With these somatics exercises, can I continue to lift weights at the gym?

A. There's nothing wrong with weightlifting as long as you practice safely and intelligently. However, keep in mind that the goals of these respective approaches, though not outright contradictory, are substantially different. Of course, not all weightlifting is the same. So, any answer I provide must consider that there are a variety of approaches to lifting weights. Because weightlifting, by design, generally isolates certain muscles, it could even be argued that lifting weights encourages muscle differentiation, though not exactly in an "intelligence promoting" manner. In truth, the way most people lift weights hardly qualifies as exercise in mindful differentiation. As a rule, there is nothing meditative or particularly integrative about pumping iron, despite the release of endorphins or the perception of stress release. Usually, weightlifting entails forceful muscular contractions that are goal-oriented and immediately gratifying, little more than a means to an end, with scant attention to any deeper internal sense of process or creative purposefulness. Weightlifting does little to promote intelligence in the muscles and may even serve to cause, reinforce, or aggravate issues of sensorimotor amnesia. This is particularly true for persons who lift for bulky muscle mass (e.g., bodybuilders) because the rate at which the body rebuilds damaged muscle tissue may exceed the rate at which that new tissue becomes innervated. The result can be, literally, stupid muscles. Of course, there are benefits to weightlifting, such as building and maintaining bone density and muscle tone. Even so, there can be a downside to pumping iron. So, the answer is: yes, you can lift weights, but at what risk?

In contrast to weightlifting, somatics is all about enhancing neuromuscular intelligence and communication. This makes somatic education an ideal co-practice for weightlifters, or for any other activity that places heavy demands on the body. Weightlifters can count on somatics to enhance innervation of rebuilt muscle tissue, which will facilitate a greater sense of differentiation both in and out of the gym. Somatics can also help weightlifters to avoid or redress chronic muscle tightness, or tendencies to same.

Q. How often should I do my somatics home exercises? And when is the best time to practice?

A. Practice your somatics movement patterns daily for best results. There's very little wiggle room on this. You need to assign your somatic movement patterns the same level of importance as brushing your teeth or changing your socks. I wouldn't lose sleep over a missed day now and then, but daily practice makes for best results.

As for when to practice, morning is probably the most beneficial time. During sleep your endocrine system releases restorative hormones (HGH, ACTH, cortisol, etc.) that repair the body where necessary, but which contribute to stiffness on waking. Think of what a cat or dog does on waking. It stretches its haunches and arches its back. This is natural for animals, as it should be for you. Mindful stretching first thing in the morning makes for a great way to start your day.

You can also benefit from doing somatics patterns before bedtime, to rid your body of any muscular stress accumulated during the day. This can be especially useful for people who have difficulty sleeping. I'd add that there's nothing wrong with "customizing" your practice, applying the principles of somatics to whatever your body is doing throughout the day. For example, I like to practice my Arch and Flatten[1] maneuver while driving in a sitting position to prevent low back tightness, or a few mindful spinal twists while engaged for any length at my computer. Keep in mind, though, that such brief interludes do not comprise an acceptable substitute for regular dedicated practice sessions. Also, interlude practice, by its very nature, can undermine the lingering mindfulness that characterizes a more relaxed and dedicated approach.

Q. I'm in my fifties and have started dating again. I'm finding that many men my age have libido or sexual dysfunction problems, or at least diminished performance. Is there anything that somatics might have to offer to help in this situation?

A. Assuming that the issue is not one of desire, and simply one of performance, somatics may indeed be of some help. Diminished libido or sexual dysfunction can be caused or abetted by a number of factors. Certainly somatics is no panacea in this regard. But if stress is implicated, or if poor circulation is at cause, then somatics, overall, and Thomas Hanna's breathing and middle body patterns in particular may prove helpful in improving performance. The somatics breathing patterns developed by Hanna are quite potent, in that they promote fuller respiration to oxygenate the blood, and serve to induce blood flow to the lower abdominal region. Before learning somatics, I practiced for many years at a particular qigong discipline that entailed breathing powerfully into the perineal region, one inadvertent effect of

---

1 Arch and Flatten is part of Lesson 1 in *The Myth of Aging* series. Further description of this movement pattern is also included in the guided movement pattern; *Movements for Sensing & Freeing the Sacrum & Cranium*; see Chapter 13.

which was to increase libido. Since learning somatics, I've found that Hanna's breathing methods closely parallel that discipline in their effects, plus they're much easier to learn.

Q. We've just spent the whole weekend learning the eight "Myth of Aging" patterns. But I don't have hours of free time every day to practice. What can I do?

A. Naturally, you can't put the rest of your life on hold while you just do somatics. Now that you've learned these patterns you have several options available. First, the Cat Stretch represents a shortened version of these exercises. Dr. Hanna excerpted the most important patterns and distilled them into a condensed format that addresses your whole body in as short a span as ten or fifteen minutes per practice session. You can find the Cat Stretch in CD format, or in Hanna's book, *Somatics*, or as a transcribed insert in many of Hanna's electronic media courses. You can also pick and choose amongst the individual movement patterns according to your perceived need. On any given day you may feel you need more hip and waist work, while on another day your neck and shoulders may call for more attention.

As you continue integrating these practices on a regular basis, your growing familiarity with them will instinctively guide you to whichever practice is best for you at any given time. Some days a ten-minute morning session will be adequate to your needs. Others days you may find that issues in your body or acute stressors call for extra time and more focused attention. Generally, the more you practice any given pattern, the more familiar it will become to your brain and body, thereby requiring progressively less practice time to remind your body how to organize and manage itself.

Q. I've been practicing Ashtanga Yoga for several years, which keeps my body fit and flexible, or so I thought. I didn't understand why I still had lower back pain until you showed me how my posture was off while standing upright. The somatics exercises relieved my back pain right away. But when I practice Somatics patterns amongst a group of people like this, I can't help but notice that most other people are a lot less flexible. You'd think that being more flexible would immediately put one at an advantage. My question is this: is there any relationship between how far you can stretch with somatics exercises and the benefits that you get from them?

A. Great question. For somebody like you, unusually fit and toned and flexible, the natural tendency may be to push your body to the limits of its range of motion, like with your yoga. However, pushing your body to its limits is not what somatics is about. If you're straining to achieve maximum flexibility you're missing within that process an important opportunity to gain better voluntary control of your muscles. You'd be better off practicing well short of your body's limits, but conducting your practice in a way (i.e., slowly and methodically) that challenges your brain's ability to control the movement at a more nuanced level. In other words, practice smaller and slower rather than bigger and faster. Remember, it is sensitivity and control of your body that you want to achieve first and foremost, even before flexibility. Flexibility and muscular intelligence are not the same. Practicing incorrectly by jerking quickly into a posture, or by pushing yourself to a point of strain contributes nothing whatsoever to your self-sensing abilities or to your neuromuscular intelligence.

Q. I definitely feel a difference after my clinical session on the table, but will it stick?

A. I'm tempted to say that's entirely up to you, contingent on your willingness to keep up with your supporting home practice patterns. The truth is, though, that factors other than your compliance in keeping up regular home practice may have some bearing on how well and how fully you retain your benefits. First, at the risk of sounding like a broken record, you have to do your home practice exercises daily, otherwise you're wasting our time and your money. Even knowing a lot about somatics is of limited value if you fail to keep up your practice. That said, lifestyle may play some role here as well. If the stressors on your body that initially caused your problems remain present in your life, you'll be waging an uphill battle. I have some clients who engage in heavy manual labor as part of their job. They inform me that doing their exercises regularly helps a lot in managing their body stress, but even so they still need to pop in every few months for a somatics "tune up."

Generally, if you reinforce the gains you've made in a clinical session with the prescribed home practice, AND you manage to avoid behaviors or experiences that would undo those gains, there should be no reason for your improvements to not stick. Significantly, as your body accustoms itself through regular practice to healthy relaxed muscles, this healthier state will become your new norm, versus any previous norm of chronic stress or tension that prompted you to try somatics.

Q. Between kids and work and all the busyness of my day I simply don't have time to practice somatics exercises every day. I mean, what happens if I don't do my exercises as prescribed? Am I wasting my time? Would I be better off trying something else to relieve my painful condition?

A. In a word or two, yes and no. Yes, it's possible you'll be wasting your time. And, no, if somatics works for you when practiced correctly, then the likelihood is that the unique approach of somatics is what best addresses your particular issues, and for good reason. If somatics is what works for you other modalities may not be similarly effective.

Let's deal with the "yes" first. To begin, how will you recognize if you're wasting your time? You'll know this when your efforts (assuming you are practicing correctly) fail to produce the desired results. As somatic educators, our policy is that you practice your movement patterns daily for best results. This is not some arbitrary homework assignment on our part. If you have sensorimotor amnesia it means your muscles have already become habituated in a certain unhealthy way. This habituation means your brain has adopted an errant default pattern for your muscles. This habituation is the root cause of your problems. To alleviate the problem you must reprogram a new (and healthy) default pattern into your brain. There is no other way around this, not if you want lasting results. HSE clinical table work and exercise patterns are designed specifically to reinforce correct neuromuscular patterns in your body. If your errant pattern is longstanding or part of a "problem complex," or if you are continually exposed to stressors that are likely to re-trigger the errant pattern, daily practice is a must. If your problems are acute and simple, and if you are unlikely to reencounter aggravating stressors, then you may be able, eventually, to wean back somewhat from every-single-day practice. You'll need to develop a sensitivity to your own body's tolerance and resilience to determine what works best for you.

As for switching to some other modality, you can't reasonably expect to reap the same benefits by substituting a different modality just because it's more convenient to your lifestyle. If the unique features of somatics are pre-cisely what your body needs, then other modalities may produce short-term improvements only, or they may cover up (palliate) a problem without fixing it. Any other modality that fails to address the underlying causes in the brain is unlikely to produce lasting improvement. A poor substitute makes for a poor strategy for living in the best way. I find somatics exercises fun and easy, and a great way to learn about myself while assuming a fuller responsibility for my own health and well-being. I suggest that you don't have time to *not* practice your exercises, even if just for a few minutes each day. Attending to your own health and wellness in the best way needs to be Job #1.

Q. I've been practicing some of these somatics exercises for a while. At first they felt great and I really felt a difference. But lately I'm not getting the same results. What gives? Have they stopped working for me?

A. When I work with clients one on one on my table I always give them home practice exercises to reinforce the changes their bodies have undergone. These exercises may be excerpts from *The Myth of Aging* series or other patterns developed by Hanna himself or other HSE teaching experts. Regardless of the exercise, and whether learned in follow-up to a clinical session or as a separate practice, the principles remain constant according to Hanna's design. In every case, the efficacy of the exercise hinges, not on the mere mechanics of the pattern, but on the manner in which it is performed. Of course, it's helpful to get the mechanics right too.

I make a point of reviewing periodically with clients those exercises I have prescribed to them on previous occasions. Not infrequently, I observe on review that clients have an inexact grasp of the pattern, requiring corrections to their practice routine. Even more often, what happens is that people get so used to doing an exercise the same way, day after day, that they relegate it to automatic pilot as they shift into rote performance. They make the error of expecting that a perfunctory execution of the movements will be adequate to produce the desired results. In doing so, people can forget that these movement patterns are only tools. They won't do anything more for you than you do for yourself with them.

The purpose of these exercises is to recover voluntary control of your muscles through conscious self-sensing. The more you use a tool, the more you become an expert craftsman. It follows that absenting your truly mindful attention on a moment-by-moment basis to what your body is doing, you can't possibly be contributing to a resumption of voluntary control (if you only go through the motions perfunctorily). It's not enough to merely do the exercise. Not to sound corny, but you must *become* the exercise to gain best results.

When it comes to somatics exercises, your perceptive attention strongly influences your reality. For example, your current reality is that you're sitting here listening to (or reading) this answer. So you're probably not paying attention while you sit to the quality of your posture or the fullness of your breath or the weight of your body on your sitting bones. With this simple reminder as you read these words, you might find yourself doing just that—you become more aware of yourself and perhaps you make adjustments to your posture—and doing so changes your reality, even if just a little bit.

It's quite true that your exercise patterns may offer some degree of benefit regardless of how correctly you perform them. But, to become masterful, like a craftsman, at managing your own body you need to pay attention at a deeper level and in a mindful manner. Note—my operative advice to you centers around *be*-ing in the moment, not *was*-ing in the moment. Mindfulness is a virtue that must be continually practiced to be of genuine value. Try going back and practicing your same movements, but practice them as if you were actively discovering and exploring them for the first time, slowly and mindfully. Try to do this each and every time you practice.

Q. I'm wondering if one of the effects of somatics is to move Qi energy in any way similar to acupuncture.

A. In determining whether somatics moves energy in any way similar to acupuncture we must first anticipate that the answer hinges on some hidden variables. So there's no simple "Yes, it does" or "No, it doesn't" response to this query. To arrive at any useful answer we must first understand something about the nature of energy. We must also distinguish between the deliberate process of moving energy and the more inadvertent *fait accompli*—that energy has been moved—in establishing wherein may lie any similarities between somatics and acupuncture.

According to traditional Chinese medicine (TCM), Qi energy that moves and expands both confers and indicates health and vibrance, even life itself. Energy that depletes and stagnates, on the other hand, is debilitating—it leads to illness and accelerates the aging process. Therefore, the most essential nature of life-force energy in living beings is to "move." Only when Qi moves, and does so freely, are human beings able to live freely. Until and unless some force or influence interferes with its natural flow, Qi moves optimally according to nature's design. Examples of interfering forces might include stress/tension/

anxiety, illness, injury/trauma, energy depletion/exhaustion, or death itself.

Acupuncture works specifically and directly to influence the flow of Qi by targeting locations in the body via known energy gates where energy can be accessed, usually near the skin's surface. Needles are inserted into these gates (points) to not only move energy, but also to regulate how it moves. Depending on what a patient requires to restore health, this could entail freeing up energy that is sluggish or modulating energy that is overactive, or otherwise adjusting according to need. How, exactly, one's energy is fine-tuned can vary according to the type of metal in the needle, or according to how the needle is manipulated after insertion, or by the point or sequence or combination of points chosen for insertion. Somatics does not seek to influence energy in this same way. However, in its more general regard, the overall purpose of acupuncture is to manipulate energy in ways that restore balance and lead to healing and maintenance of the patient. In this more general regard an argument might be made that somatics is similar.

Somatics is not overtly geared toward moving energy. Rather, somatics is more designed to restore voluntary control to muscles that have become compromised due to sensorimotor amnesia, which may or may not be causatively linked to the body's energy system. "Moving energy" is inevitably concomitant to the more direct intent of somatics because muscles that are in a compromised state must also suffer from some degree of energy dissonance. But, just how profound the impact of the somatics restorative process is on the body's energy system may vary according to factors having little to do with somatics as a treatment modality.

I believe somatics is no more akin to acupuncture than it is to chiropractic, or yoga, or Tai Chi, or a long soak in a hot tub for that matter...which is to say it can be somewhat similar. Any therapy that produces a change in the organism must also have some effect on its energy. To what degree is that effect? To what degree is it genuinely therapeutic? And to what degree is it durably ameliorative versus merely palliative? Again, that depends.

If you accept the basic premise of what I have already noted, it follows that the process of restoring voluntary control to compromised muscles—which, themselves, have been chronically engaged and less able to move freely—can't *not* have a collateral effect on the energy systems proximate to the muscles in question. However, the therapeutic value and the long-term efficacy of the experience may vary according to the etiology and the extent of involvement. If a muscle is in distress and if that distress is due to an energetic cause, then addressing the muscle (even if the treatment is "successful") is unlikely to produce an appreciable improvement in the flow of energy because the underlying cause remains unaddressed. What's more, the long-term efficacy of the somatics effect may be in jeopardy and the problem prone to recurrence if the causative factors (the energy imbalance) remain unaddressed. However, if the energy imbalance is incidental to another cause, e.g., trauma to the muscle stemming from causes not attributable to an energy imbalance, then addressing the muscle with somatics may restore energy flow. In this case somatics will have addressed the underlying cause. In the first case attending to the muscle somatically may, de facto, be less similar to acupuncture because restoration of muscle function may have a negligible effect on collateral energy function. In the second case, the exact same somatic approach may restore energy flow to its optimal state. It all depends on whether the somatics approach addresses the underlying cause of the problem or merely one of its expressions.

As mentioned, energy will necessarily be caused to move by any somatic session, even if incidental. How directly that energy mobilization will be involved in any healing response—whether it facilitates a healing response, or moves in consequence to a healing response—depends also on the nature of the pathology. In answer to the question posed, I'd suggest the less inadvertent the patient's energetic response to any somatics session, the more somatics might be said to move energy in a way similar to acupuncture.

I also believe that the subjective intention of any practitioner can influence the efficacy of a treatment (though more likely from an energetic perspective than from a musculoskeletal perspective). The same acupuncture needle inserted into the same acupuncture point by two different practitioners may have a variable effect. Perhaps the effect might not be so marked in the case of two equally skilled acupuncturists. But a less-experienced practitioner may not achieve the same result, even with the same insertion point, as a practitioner who is masterful at his craft to a point of being able to augment the effects of a needle with his own energy. Because somatics presents as a relatively more mechanical and less energetic discipline than acupuncture, the role of the practitioner's intention (as distinct from technical mastery or a good bedside manner) is probably less influential in the client's healing response.

All that said, and though this is an interesting academic question, my inclination is to leave the practice of deliberate "energy work" to those providers best trained in that approach.

Q. I'd like to know what you think about somatics and emotions. After my last clinical session I was driving home and I experienced a powerful release of emotions. Do you think there might any connection between the two?

A. Quite probably, yes. This is something I wrote about in an earlier book (*Exploring Tai Chi*). I observed over four decades of teaching martial arts that many people are predominantly of the mind or of the body. People who are first and foremost of the mind experience new information cognitively before trying to apply what they've learned with their bodies. People who are predominantly of the body opt for direct experience first, as a basis for trying to make sense of that experience in their heads. An example can be seen in two hypothetical individuals who each enter into psychotherapy. The first patient, being someone of the mind, proceeds easily in accessing feelings and talking out issues, even issues having to do with body management. But when she then goes to yoga class, or for golf lessons, or any other such physical activity she presents as a bit out of her element, perhaps not at all outstanding as a natural athlete. Meanwhile, the second counseling patient, who is more of the body, struggles mightily while in therapy to access genuine feelings or self-assessments. After therapy he goes for a run, or plays sports or mows the lawn, and while actively engaged at "doing something" he finds himself achieving the very reflections and insights that were just shortly ago, in the context of a more corticalized talk therapy, just out of reach. Kids make for an even simpler scenario. Some kids will predictably dive into new activities headlong, while others need to process things a bit first before getting involved.

If you are a "body person," the release of longstanding muscular tensions that often accompanies a session in somatics can certainly produce a commensurate release, or processing, of pent-up emotions. This certainly makes one more compelling reason to practice somatics at all times in a slow and purposeful fashion, lest the momentum of perfunctory practice preclude the release or expression of emotions or insights that may be percolating below the surface. Conversely, if you tend to be more of the mind, the slow purposefulness of your practice may better enable you to experience your own body in ways previously less attainable.

Q. Given all I've heard about the similarities and compatibility between Taijiquan and somatics, I'm wondering if Tai Chi might be regarded as an early form of somatics?

A. Cute question. I'd have to say in answer, "no" and "perhaps."

I say "no" first of all because somatics is somatics, and Taijiquan is Taijiquan. Also, despite the similarities, there are many disparities between the two disciplines. Somatics is a modality solidly rooted in neurophysiology, the purpose of which is to elicit a specific kind of neurological recalibration in preventing or redressing pathological neuromuscular habituation. Tai Chi, on the other hand, concerns itself, among other features, with managing Qi energy and, notably, with martial application, which are two important aspects not present in somatics.

However, I say "perhaps" because Tai Chi, like somatics, relies on the body as the primary medium to achieve a congruent philosophical existence, one based on achieving and living from the perspective of freedom of mind and body. In weighing the more profound philosophical parallels of Tai Chi and somatics against several of the more practical means by which their respective ends are met, I have to admit the parallels seem to outweigh the divergences, as in "all roads lead to Rome."

So, in a generalized sense, I suppose Tai Chi could be construed as an early cousin, if not a direct forerunner, of HSE. I will go out on a limb here in noting the theoretical similarity of somatics also to many of the different qigong practices that I have learned and practiced over the last several decades. Many of the qualities so defining to certain qigong methods—purposeful breathing, mindful attention to process, being in the moment, and articulate positionings and manueverings of the body in specific or exacting postures—are substantively akin to somatics. On a practical level, I encourage all my Taijiquan and qigong students to learn somatics to better master their respective disciplines.

All attempts at categorizing aside, there is no doubt that we have in somatics and Taijiquan two approaches to personal wellness that share many similarities and offer the prospect of being mutually complementary. Incidentally, judging by what I've heard of his archived lectures, Thomas Hanna was well familiar with Tai Chi and seemed to hold this ancient art in high regard. Perhaps his exposure to Tai Chi even influenced Hanna's thinking in ways we can only speculate about.

Q. I'm interested in finding out about undertaking a study of somatics toward earning certification as a practitioner, not for myself but for my son who is a chiropractor. However, I'm a little uncertain about your business model. How can anyone make any money if they're only seeing clients on such a short-term basis?

A. I appreciate your being so candid with your concerns. You've raised a very interesting economic and ethical question. Namely, how can somatics practitioners make a living plying their trade if their clients achieve the sought-after results in a mere several sessions? To be financially successful any healing practice needs to strike some balance between clients who return for services on a regular and predictable basis and an ongoing supply of new clients to continually refresh a diminished client base. How many people do you know who have been receiving long-term therapeutic care without really getting or staying better? I'd be circumspect about therapeutic practices that are heavily dependent on clients to continually return for ongoing services. Why aren't those clients staying better?

In somatics, our goal as educators is (ideally) to resolve clients' issues and discharge them in three–five sessions (or less), whenever possible. So it seems fair to say that somatics practices are more predicated on attracting new clients versus having the same old clients coming back forever. Unfortunately, having a broad base for potential new clients is not much of a problem for us because neuromuscular distress is fairly rampant, something that most people suffer from. On a more positive note, the resolution of sensorimotor amnesia is our particular area of expertise, so in this regard somatics is often effective where other modalities are not.

I have to admit that without clients continually returning for services on a long term basis, the onus does fall on each somatic practitioner to attract new clients. We have our work cut out for us in educating the public as to the relative pros and cons of somatics. So, at least until somatics becomes more of a household word, a successful practice must rely on marketing and education, as well as referrals, so people can understand why they would seek out a somatic educator. Usually, there's no shortage of referrals from happy clients.

As with any other business, there are other practical considerations, aside from any individual practitioner's skill level, that will determine financial success or failure. Is the practice located in an urban, suburban, or rural setting? How effective are the practitioner's business skills? What is the business overhead? Is the practice full-time or part-time? And so on. In my practice, I schedule clients as time allows, which is to say when I'm not otherwise engaged at writing books or teaching martial arts. Some of my colleagues see a few clients a week. Others maintain a full-time practice with a waiting list. The financial success of any practice hinges on quite a number of variables. But I believe if a practitioner is skilled and can help people live more rewarding and pain-free lives, clients will come.

From an ethical perspective, it's our job as somatic educators to help clients resolve those issues that brought them to us as quickly and as fully as possible. Plus, at a societal level, somatics can offer a quick and relatively inexpensive means of addressing at least one part of our national healthcare crisis, to ease the burden on our nation's healthcare system. Financial considerations aside, I find my contribution in both these respects to be very gratifying.

PART 4

SOMATIC MOVEMENT PATTERNS

CHAPTER 13

SENSING AND FREEING
THE SACRUM AND CRANIUM

Movements for Sensing and Freeing the Sacrum and Cranium

The following is a comprehensive example of one in a series of somatic movement patterns composed by the author. There are many such patterns and series of patterns, arranged thematically according to somatic conditions or by body area, e.g., Delicate Backs, Protruding Bellies, Full Breathing, etc. This lesson series, as well as an expansive selection of others, are available in CD format.[1] The vast majority of somatics narratives were recorded by HSE founder Thomas Hanna. Without exception, Hanna's narratives present extraordinary learning opportunities worth exploring.

Note: Where the directions indicate for a "Pause and practice," exercise your own best discretion in allotting whatever time you feel is appropriate or comfortable before continuing on.

Lesson 1

The following includes a series of lessons designed to guide you in enhancing your understanding and control of the muscles governing the movement of your lower back and upper spine and neck areas. To derive an optimal benefit from these teachings, it is important to learn and practice them in a context free from distraction. Finding a firm yet comfortable padded surface, such as a mat or a carpet on the floor, will ensure best results. Each

---

1 Thomas Hanna's guided movement patterns are also available in cassette format.

lesson is approximately ten to twenty minutes in length, though the time you spend can vary according to your inclination to linger or move along. The purpose of these movements is not to exercise, condition, or strengthen your body in the manner of popular fitness workouts. Rather, all movements are to be done having in mind the idea of sensing and experiencing fully the differentiation of the muscular nuances involved, as well the interplay between your intention, your self-awareness, and your breath.

Practice: Begin by lying on your back with your knees drawn up. Position your feet flat with your heels comfortably close to your buttocks. For readers not already familiar with the Arch and Flatten sequence, inhale gently into your abdomen as you simultaneously arch your lower back upward from the floor. Your pelvis should not break contact with the floor. Instead, you'll want your sacroiliac (pelvis) to roll gently downward along the sacrum[2] as if you were trying to touch your tailbone (coccyx) to the floor. Then, as you slowly exhale your breath, roll back up along the sacrum, lifting your tailbone away from the floor and flattening the beltline portion of your lower back down firmly. You want to feel your line of contact against the floor moving up along the back of your pelvis, from your tailbone to the upper crest of your sacrum. Throughout, your pelvis should move like a rolling pin against the floor. Repeat this arching and flattening sequence a few times on your own, moving slowly and breathing with a sense of deliberate awareness to the muscle functions involved. Pause and practice.

Reflections: Stop and rest for just a moment to give both your body and your mind a chance to digest what you've just done. This simple pattern represents one essential feature in maintaining a healthy and balanced body. Arching your lower back upwards in a manner that is coordinated with your breath calls into play the Landau reflex, a primitive reflex mechanism that

---

2   Your sacrum is the large triangular bone at the lower end of your spine housed within the pelvic girdle. The coccyx trails off the lower end of the sacrum.

first makes its appearance in humans at about four or five months of age. Before the onset of this reflex, infants can only flex forward into a fetal curve. It is the onset of this arching reflex that activates the body's most central extensor muscles and facilitates lifting of one's head, standing upright and, eventually, walking forward into one's destiny. Conversely, flattening your lower back down against the floor as you exhale activates your most central flexors, muscles that are typically called into play as one part of the body's sympathetic reflex action known as the Startle Response. Both of these reflex patterns are necessary to a healthy and optimally functioning body. Either or both of them can be problematic, however, if the muscles associated with the action become so chronically habituated that they lose their ability to fully relax when your brain is not calling them into play.

As you proceed into your movement pattern, and throughout these exercises, try to imagine your body as a map laid out flat on the floor, and that your vantage has you looking down at your body from above. Imagining your body as a map will help you to organize according to a directional context. Upward, toward your head, will be north. Downward, toward your feet, is south. Your left side (remember, your left side will appear to your right when viewed from above) will be designated as east, and your right side as west [Figure 13-1].

Practice: Resume your arching and flattening, paying special attention to the top-to-bottom axis along which your sacrum is rolling in its contact against the floor. Try to feel and identify the lowest, or southernmost, point where your tailbone touches down. This will occur as your lower back (approximately at the level of your beltline) arches up and away from the floor. Pause momentarily. Now, gradually flatten your lower back as you exhale, and try to feel and identify the highest, or northernmost, point where the upper ridge of your sacrum touches down. Pause briefly. Continue to roll your sacrum alternately upward and downward to develop a familiarity with the vertical axis running between your uppermost contact point at the sacrum and the lowermost contact point at your coccyx. Practice this up-and-down movement several times. Pause and practice.

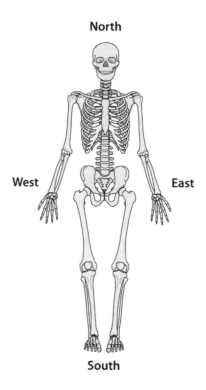

North

West

East

South

Figure 13-1. Looking down at your body from above.

Next, try to pinpoint what feels to you like the exact midpoint between these two polar opposites. Pause, and hold your sacrum steady at this midpoint as you prepare to establish a horizontal axis, perpendicular to your already-established vertical axis. Think of this new perpendicular axis as the equator to your north/south longitudinal line. Shift your weight east along this equator line to the leftmost side of your sacrum. Slowly, move your weight back and forth along this line between your center point and east. Try this several times on your own to get a good feel for it, and then settle back at your center. Pause and practice.

Now, shift west along your equator line to the right. Again, move between your center point and west a few times on your own, familiarizing yourself with this new terrain. Pause and practice.

Next, shift back and forth on your sacroiliac between east and west. Notice for any differences between the two sides. Pause and practice.

Return to your central point where the two axes intersect and again move up and down along your north/south axis a few times. Pause and practice.

Lie still and rest.

Reflections: The basic idea here is to notice everything you can possibly notice about whatever it is you're doing, in this case working in a precisely articulate manner in maneuvering the central regions of your body. The movement patterns, themselves, can be beneficial, but your greatest benefits will stem from your careful attention to the underlying processes.

Under normal circumstances, the filtering mechanisms of your brain highlight for conscious scrutiny only those experiences or awarenesses which warrant priority status, for example, "Are you hungry? And, if so, where's your next meal coming from?" or, "How are you placing your feet or steering your car as you walk along an icy pavement?" These are issues of immediate concern to your brain's sense of health and well-being. Meanwhile, millions of other lessor concerns, among which might be the specific muscles involved in that chronic tightness in your lower back, tend to be screened out of conscious awareness. Such less-pressing stimuli are relegated to an amorphous background, such as when your back is habitually tight or restricted, but not yet at a level that's commanding your attention with acute pain.

Just as with Tai Chi, the slower you move your body the more opportunity you have to notice important, but generally amorphous, aspects of your own being. In the noticing you gain the ability to differentiate and recover a fuller voluntary control over those same aspects, to reclaim them as it were from the amorphous realm. As you improve your ability to notice and control, so will you improve both your proprioceptive literacy and sensorimotor functioning. These are important and necessary steps on your path to personal mastery and optimal musculoskeletal health.

Practice: Resume by rolling your sacrum to flatten your back down, so that its northernmost contact point is touching against the floor. From here, you're will establish a second horizontal axis across the top of your sacrum, exactly parallel to your equator line. Shift along the top of your sacrum to the left so that you're touching down at the northeastern-most point. Move back and forth a few times between north-center and northeast. Pause and practice.

Reverse, and shift back in the opposite direction, exploring between north-center and northwest. Pause and practice.

Slowly move back and forth across the full width of this horizontal axis, differentiating northeast from northwest, and differentiating the whole of this axis from the axis below, at your equator. Pause and practice.

Come back to north center and roll down again to your exact midpoint, and from that midpoint, continue to roll further down on your sacrum to its southernmost point, where you will establish a third horizontal axis. Do the same here as above, exploring slowly between south-center and southeast.

Slowly, do the same between south-center and southwest. Pause and practice.

Practice going back and forth, between left and right, across the full width of your lower sacrum.

Take a few moments and experiment, moving sideways along each of these three axes in turn. Feel for subtle differences between the three, as well as for any referred sensations or awarenesses in the surrounding muscles of your lower back, or in your shoulders, or anywhere else in your body. Pause and practice.

Return to your central position. Lay flat and rest for a full minute or so.

To resume, position your sacrum at its southernmost point. Having already established two additional horizontal axes parallel to your original equator, you will now enact similar reference lines vertically. Starting from being weighted at your lower left sacrum, shift your weight upwards along left to the upper left, or northeastern aspect of your sacrum. Shift slowly up and down along the eastern axis of your sacrum several times. Pause and practice.

Settle your sacrum back at southeast. From here, shift along the lower rim of your sacrum to the lower right, to your southwestern-most aspect. Now move in the same manner, from southwest to northwest, up and down along your western axis. Do this several times, then lay flat and relax.

Reflections: The sacroiliac area, in back, is nothing more than one side of that coin we call the waist. Your waist serves as a "transfer station" of sorts for all the forces that traverse between your upper body and your lower body, acting much like a power transformer. This is to say that just about anything you do calls into service the muscles of your waist and lower back. Given the usual unhealthy demands that people put on these muscles, it's no surprise that most people are likely to experience lower back pain, or pain referred to some other area but stemming from their lower back, as they go through life. Articulating your sacrum in a manner such as you are learning here—one that includes deliberate attention to these very muscles—affords you a means by which you can incrementally regain fuller voluntary control over the central regions of your body to avoid or manage the discomforts and inconveniences of lower back pain.

Practice: Let's take what you've learned so far and arrange your movements according to a specific pattern. Move slowly at first in implementing this new pattern. Bring your attention to your sacrum at its southeastern-most corner. Shift on your sacrum to the right, at southwest, and from there, roll directly up along the sacrum to northwest. From northwest, shift directly left across to northeast, and roll south, back to your starting point at southeast. Continue in this manner, exercising careful control in tracing out with your sacrum a square or rectangular pattern. Practice this, at first, in a clockwise direction. Pause and practice.

Begin to trace your pattern just a little faster, noticing how you inevitably round the corners of your square as the tracing movements of your sacrum quicken. You'll notice that your square increasingly comes to resemble a circle. After a few times around, gradually slow your pace until you ease to a stop. Rest for a moment.

Resume your pattern, but now in exactly the opposite direction. Begin at southeast and roll up to northeast. Shift across to northwest, and roll down to southwest. Complete your counterclockwise pattern by shifting across to southeast. Continue tracing out your square, and after a few repetitions gradually convert this square into a circle as you pick up the pace just a bit. Pause and practice.

Slow your movement and bring your tracing to a halt. Rest comfortably as you breathe slowly and consciously into your lower abdomen. This completes Lesson 1.

Reminder: Practice each lesson as many times as it takes until your practice feels comfortable and smooth, before advancing to the next lesson. Remember, progress is measured not in how quickly you advance to the next lesson, but in how thoroughly you integrate what you've learned. There's no rush.

Lesson 2

Practice: To begin, lay down on your back and review, a few times on your own, the Arch and Flatten movements covered in Lesson 1. As you practice this pattern, remember that your full and curious attention to the inner nuances of each movement is much more important than any concern you might give to the number of repetitions or to any aspect of satisfaction at feeling as though you've given yourself a good workout. Softness and awareness take precedence in these practices over expediency and exertion. Pause and practice.

Thus far, you have learned how to articulate your sacrum in a grid, along a series of vertical and horizontal axes, and also in square and circular maneuvers. I'd like for you to try something new at this stage.

Begin by shifting onto your lower right sacrum, at the southwest. From here, you are going to establish a new corridor. Shift on your sacrum diagonally up and across to its center, and then continue on diagonally to the upper left, at northeast [Figure 13-2, line A]. Practice moving your sacrum up and down along this diagonal corridor. Notice how your body adjusts to this new articulation in a manner slightly, or perhaps even quite noticeably, different from when it was moving straight up and down or across. Pay attention, in particular, for changes in the shifting of weight at your lower back, waist, and shoulders. Pause and practice. [Note: Figures 13-2, 13-3, and 13-4 each offer frontal views of how to organize movements at the back of your sacroiliac area.]

Shift to the lower left and apply the same model along the opposite diagonal corridor, between lower left and upper right [Figure 13-2, line B]. Pause and practice.

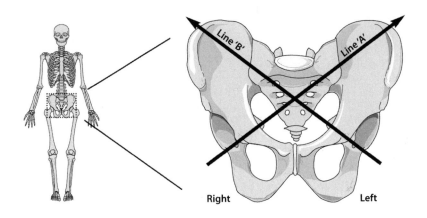

Figure 13-2. Diagonal corridors.

Let's indulge in something a bit more creative. This next part is optional, but if you feel comfortable with what you've done so far you can try moving your sacrum in a Figure 8. Starting from your lower left, at southeast, move diagonally to the upper right...and from there horizontally across to your upper left...then diagonally down to your lower right...horizontally back across to your lower left, and so on [Figure 13-3]. This may take some concentration at first. Moving slowly, very slowly, is the key, and the means by which you will develop the muscular differentiation and control necessary to complete the intricacies of this movement pattern. Pause and practice.

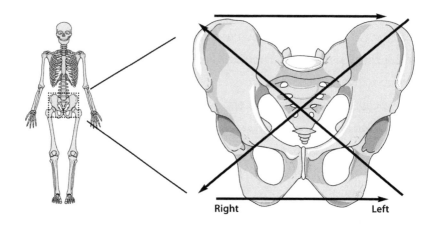

Right   Left

Figure 13-3. Figure 8 pattern.

Come to a stop and rest while you digest this new level of learning. In moving through your Figure 8, I've directed you in moving in one direction only. After you've rested a bit you can try experimenting on your own with reversing the direction of your Figure 8 pattern.

Reflections: Think about what you've accomplished thus far through these lessons, and the extent of control that in just a brief time you have come to exercise over a part of your body you probably never thought to try maneuvering in such a controlled manner. Your ability to experience and enjoy your body as being truly free is entirely contingent on your being able to exercise voluntary control over your body. Freedom and control, along with differentiation, go hand in hand. You cannot, after all, control what you can't differentiate. The experience of working this deeply within may be entirely new for you and feel daunting at first. Keep in mind that the territory you're now charting is within yourself, and so the charting process is always within your control.

To initiate change, any change, it is incumbent upon each of us to assume a certain risk in taking a first step, as you now have, in acting on a particular belief—in this case the most basic belief that you CAN change. In taking this first step and the steps that follow, you are consciously and unconsciously assuming a new level of responsibility for how you live your life. You are asserting control over yourself to become freer. So far, we have confined the focus of attention primarily to a small area at the center of your physical self. The idea of slowing down to pay attention for details that are already present, to achieve differentiation and personal control and the freedom that ensues, is a concept that can be applied at every level of your life.

Practice: Let's try one final pattern to complete this level of learning. This exercise will seem challenging at first and will require exacting precision in controlling the muscles of your sacrum and pelvis as well as those of your waist and lower back. In moving your sacrum according to your several vertical, horizontal, and diagonal corridors, it may have occurred to you to imagine your sacrum and pelvis as organized like a tic-tac-toe grid. Visualize your sacrum as divided into nine equal sections, three boxes wide by three boxes high [Figure 13-4]. Settle your sacrum onto its middle-most box, the midpoint of which is exactly where your two central axes intersect. Begin to move your sacrum in a miniature clockwise circle *within the confines of this middle box*. Repeat this circling pattern several times. Pause and practice. After a few repetitions pause and reverse your circle to the opposite direction. After several repetitions pause and rest.

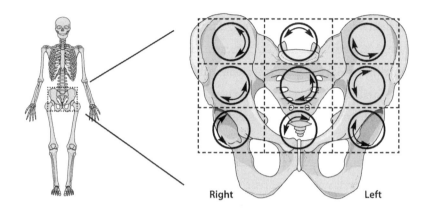

Figure 13-4. Mini circles, ala tic-tac-toe grid.

However challenging your tiny-circle-in-the-box exercise may have felt, let's shift your focus down to the box immediately below. Staying within the confines of your new box, again rotate your sacrum in the tiniest of clockwise circles. Pause. Now reverse your direction. Rest a moment.

Move your attention to the southwestern-most box, at your lower right. Repeat the same pattern, a few tiny circles clockwise, and then pause and reverse your direction to circle counterclockwise. Rest a moment.

Move your attention to the westernmost box, at mid-right. Take a few moments and repeat the same pattern. Rest a moment.

Move your attention to the northwestern-most box, at your upper right and repeat as before. Rest a moment.

Move your attention to the uppermost box, in the middle. Repeat. Rest.

Move your attention to the northeastern-most box, at your upper left. Repeat the same pattern.

Move your attention to the easternmost box, at mid-left. Repeat the same pattern. Rest a moment.

Finally, shift your attention to the southeastern-most box at your lower left. Repeat the same pattern, tiny circles first in one direction, then the other without moving outside the lines.

After completing this series of tiny circles in each of these boxes you've earned an intermission. Lie still and relax for a few minutes before standing up to move about; feel for any newfound sense of discrimination in your body as you walk. This completes Lesson 2.

Lesson 3

Practice: Start by lying on your back as we commence your third lesson in the nuances of cranial-sacral articulation. Bring your knees up to a bent position and review the Arch and Flatten pattern, putting yourself through six–ten repetitions of this pattern. After the first several repetitions divide your attention by shifting part of your awareness to notice whatever may going on away from the area of your primary lower back arch. You may notice that there is more than one arch occurring aside from what's going on in your lower back. Pay particular attention to the cervical area at the back of your neck. Try to feel the movement that occurs in your neck as you arch and flatten your lower back. There is an inverse correlation between the arch of your lower back and that along the back of your neck. As your lower back arches upward, your chin tucks slightly forward and the back of your neck moves flatter against the floor. As you flatten your lower back, your chin tilts up toward the ceiling and your neck arches slightly up and away from the floor.

Continue this movement, as you begin to transfer the greater focus of your attention from your lower spine to its uppermost portions, near where your spine and cranium meet, and from there on up along the back of your skull. Feel how the back of your head gently nods up, and then down, along the floor in a manner similar to that of your sacrum in the previous lessons. Feel, how this makes for yet another vertical axis, with the contact-against-the-floor line at the back of your head running from the center of your occiput (base of the skull) up along the occipital bone, and extending almost to the parietal bone to establish a vertical center line. Pause and practice.

Let your head come to rest at the bottom-most point of that axis, at the center of your occipital ridge. Gently nod your head up again to clearly identify where the back of your head touches the floor at its highest contact point. Roll your head up and down along this axis a few times, familiarizing yourself with the full length of the movement so that, just as with your sacrum previously, you can position your head at the exact midpoint between these two extremes. Settle your head at that midpoint, and begin to anticipate in your mind how it might feel to shift your head from left to right, back and forth.

Reflections: Before taking any further action, pay close attention at this juncture in our practice to establish an important distinction. It will be quite possible to move your head along this next horizontal axis in either of two ways. I'll guide you in moving one of these ways only. Recall how, in shifting your sacrum from side to side in our earlier sessions, I asked you to keep your knees positioned upright toward the ceiling throughout your movement. Had you allowed your knees to flop over to either side during that movement, the effects of those moves on your body would have been quite different.

Here also, with your head, let's ensure that you are moving precisely in a predetermined manner. Rather than allowing your head to roll from side to side, as if the back of your head were round like a ball (which of course it is), be careful to keep the plane of your face—your eyes and your nose—oriented upward, just as you did with your knees in our earlier sessions, so that the back of your head glides or shifts, rather than rolls, from side to side. Another way you might think of this is as if someone were using their hands to stabilize your head while shifting it for you from side to side. With this distinction in mind, visualize shifting your head, slowly and deliberately, along the central horizontal axis at the back of your head between left and right.

Practice: Begin to enact what you've been visualizing. Practice this now.
After several repetitions, bring your head back to its vertical midpoint, and just slightly tilt your chin upward, so that the back of your head touches

the floor at its highest contact point. Maintaining your eyes and nose oriented upward toward the ceiling, shift your head along this upper horizontal line to the left, and from there back across to the right. Be careful to avoid any strain in your neck muscles. Pause and practice this several times.

Return to the center and shift your head downward, so that you can feel your chin tucking in just a bit and the back of your head touching the floor at its lowest contact point, at or near the occiput. Here you can establish a third horizontal axis as you shift your head to the left, and from there across to the right, back and forth. Pause and practice.

Stop and settle the back of your head to its lower left, the equivalent of what at your sacrum we labeled as southeast. Keeping to the left, maneuver your head back and up, until it settles at northeast. When moving up and down along this vertical line you will roll your head, versus shifting it. Practice a few times before settling back at southeast.

Next, move your head horizontally from southeast across to southwest at your lower right, and from there, roll your head up along the right to northwest. Practice a few times, moving your head up and down along this vertical axis. Pause.

Reposition your head to your upper right, at northwest, and from there trace out a square pattern in a clockwise direction (as if looking down at yourself from above). Move your head left across to northeast, down to southeast, across to southwest, and back up to northwest. Trace along this square pattern several times. Pause and practice.

Begin to pick up your pace just the slightest bit, and feel the corners of your square morphing to a circular pattern. Pay attention throughout to the nuances of muscular involvement in your neck, in your shoulders, and elsewhere in your body. Pause and practice.

Slow to a stop and begin, slowly, to reverse the direction of your rotation, just as you did earlier at your sacrum. Pause and practice.

Stop and rest for a moment. Conclude this lesson by reviewing several repetitions of your Arch and Flatten movement, as per earlier instructions, observing as you do so for any feelings of enhanced sensory awareness. This concludes Lesson 3.

Lesson 4

Reflections: Begin by lying flat on your back as we begin our fourth and final installment in this learning series. Thomas Hanna was fond of calling his learning sessions "visitations." A "visit" entails going to some place other than where you typically reside, for the purpose of a new experience. The word "experience" suggests both a sensory component and the acquisition of knowledge. Were you to visit any place as a person having sensory impairment, your experience would necessarily be limited because you would be unable to process data via the absent or compromised senses. You can only have an experience of that which you are able to experience. Therefore, an important part of what you are accomplishing via these learnings is *an increase in your ability to experience*, by focusing your attention correctly for best results.

Consider, for example, that throughout your practice up to this point I have asked you to press various skeletal aspects down against the floor. You might think of these aspects as reference points, and even feel a heightened awareness to these areas (which is certainly a step in the right direction). If your focus is limited to just these reference points you may get good results in alleviating this symptom or problem or that. However, the learning you gain will be limited. If, in addition, you also adjust your awareness to pay close attention to the muscles that alternately contract and release as the *means whereby* you press into these skeletal reference points you will gain the added benefit of sensory motor awareness and differentiation. You will increase your ability to experience and learn more fully. You will be learning how to learn and, by extension, expanding your options to live more fully as a human being. The level at which you choose to pay attention makes all the difference.

"Visitation" makes for an apt description of these learning sessions as you reinforce your potential for direct and conscious sensorimotor experience and differentiation. In this series of learnings, you are exploring deeply inward and sensing for awarenesses of what your body has to offer, and so gaining some better understanding of how to control your body in the best way.

Practice and Reflection: Raise your knees up to a bent position and review your arch and flatten sequence slowly a few times on your own. Pause and practice.

Next, review rotating your sacrum in a circular clockwise direction several times, just as you learned in Lesson 1. Practice. Then reverse for several rotations counterclockwise.

Rest for a moment and reflect on if and how rotating your sacrum feels more manageable now as compared to your initial attempts. Reflection such as this can provide some standard of measure in assessing and appreciating the true value of these learnings as you continue to improve through practice over time. Note: if it already feels easier, that means you have already learned something of genuine value.

Practice: Shift your attention to the back of your head. Relying on the same model used previously for your sacrum, circle the back of your head against the floor (once again using a gliding action when moving sideways and a rolling action when moving between top and bottom). Do this three times clockwise, and then three times counterclockwise. Rest a moment.

Recalling the image of a tic-tac-toe grid, apply that imagery to the back of your head. Visualize the back of your cranium as gridded into nine roughly equal sections, or boxes, three across and three deep. The tiny-circle-in-the-box exercise that you previously experimented with at your sacrum will surely feel even more challenging as you attempt to apply it at the back of your head. Nevertheless, try to move your head slowly while staying within the confines of each individual box as you rotate the back of your head in the tiniest of circles. Begin at your center point in the middle box and, with the utmost precision, begin to trace out miniature clockwise circles. Circle three times clockwise...then reverse your direction. Try this on your own. Rest a moment.

Bring your attention to your bottom center box (near your occiput), and repeat. Rest.

Reposition to the lower right box and repeat the same pattern. Rest.

Move your attention to the westernmost box (at mid-right). Repeat the same pattern. Rest.

Move your attention to your upper right. Repeat the same pattern. Rest.

Next, move your attention to the uppermost box (at the middle). Repeat the same pattern. Rest.

Shift your attention down to the box at your upper left, and repeat. Rest.

Move your attention to the easternmost box (at mid-left). Repeat the same pattern, clockwise and then counterclockwise. Rest.

Finally, move your attention to the box at your lower left, repeating the same clockwise/counterclockwise rotation. As you complete this final pattern, lie still and relax for a few moments, allowing your body and your mind to fully digest the intricacies of this new learning.

Reflection: Were you able to notice the overlap in learning experiences between these several lessons as you practiced at this most recent pattern?

Practice: Dispensing for the moment with your secondary variety of fine and tiny circles, rotate the back of your head again according to its larger circular pattern in a clockwise direction, tracing along its uppermost, lowermost, and left and right parameters. Try to move slowly, and expand your attention to include noticing elsewhere in your body. Observe that while your head rolls according to its circles above, your sacrum below tends to move automatically and in tandem with your cranium. This likely has been going on all along but escaped your conscious awareness until you were asked to notice for it. Stop and reverse the direction of your head and notice how your sacrum changes its direction as well. Pause and rest.

Let's have you experiment with another differentiation. Move your sacrum only, from side to side, keeping your head stationary while you do so. Notice how your lower spine twists more with your sacrum, relative to your upper spine, which twists less. Pause and practice.

Now hold your sacrum still as you shift just your head from side to side. Notice how your upper spine, including your neck, participates in this movement to a much greater degree than your lower spine. Pause and practice.

Set aside, just for the moment, the care you have been exercising in gliding your cranium from side to side; and, for the sake of comparison, allow your head to fully roll from side to side, like a ball. Feel how this exaggerated turning of the head engages the upper spine even more so than gliding. Pause and practice.

Return to your gliding model and shift both your head and your sacrum simultaneously to the left. Then shift both your head and your sacrum to the right, and back and forth. Notice how the entire length of your spine rotates along with the sacrum and cranium, like an axle that is rigidly attached between two rolling wheels. Pause and practice.

Now try to shift only your cranium to the left while you simultaneously shift only your sacrum to the right. Pause. Try the reverse, moving these two components again in opposite directions. Notice the effect on your spine, and feel how this twisting pattern wrings your spine like a dishrag. This effect can be felt even more clearly if you allow your head to roll from side to side like a ball, while shifting on the sacrum. Try it a few times. Now, lie still and relax for a bit.

One final segment here: Position your sacrum onto its upper right, or northwestern, aspect. Simultaneously position your cranium on its lower right aspect. Pay close attention and double check to confirm that you've got this correct—below, at your sacrum, you have your upper right touching; and above, at your cranium, you touch with your lower right, so that the distance on your right side between your sacrum and cranium is at its shortest. Notice that one effect of this positioning is to bow your spine inward and away from the right and outward and toward the left as your whole right side is drawn into contraction. Take note that in drawing the right side of your body shorter, your left side becomes lengthened. Inhale as you simultaneously roll your sacrum down and around to its lowest point in the middle, and the back of your head up and around to its highest point at the middle. The full span of your back, including your neck, will arch up slightly as you enact this transition. Continue, shifting your sacrum across and around to its upper left aspect and your head across and around to its lower left position. Feel your spine bowed now toward the right and inward from the left as your left side is now drawn shorter.

Practice this sequence back and forth very slowly, noticing for the inverse relationship between the two sides of your body, one side shortening so that the other side can lengthen. Feel how the positioning of your sacrum and your cranium each contribute to the bowing of your spine and to the alternating contraction and lengthening of either side of your body. It is almost universally the case that in order for any one part of your body to lengthen, another corresponding part must shorten, and vice versa. Lay still and completely relax for a few moments.

Reflections: It is only natural that, as you first gain any kind of new knowledge, your attention will be narrowly focused on the learning immediately at hand. It is only after time and with continued practice that the proficiency you gain will enable you to experience your learnings both in an increasingly detailed manner, and at the same time more globally in context to all the other knowledge you already possess. In other words, the more you practice these learnings the more you stand to gain as their effects become more thoroughly integrated. Keep in mind also that the effects of these practices, and the freedom you gain, will be cumulative as you continue your practice over time. This concludes this Lesson 4.

Postscript

I want to illustrate the possibilities for how you might continue to develop your practice of this work on your own. As with Tai Chi, and with many other methods for optimizing human potential, the slower and deeper your exploration, the more all-encompassing your understanding and grasp of your practice will become. In fact, real depth work—continually mining and refining the same old learnings for new understandings and perspectives—is one of the secrets to advancing one's level of mastery at Taijiquan. So it is with somatics. For all the depth and complexity of the teachings presented herein, the benefits that may yet be gained are limited only by your own imagination and perseverance.

By way of illustration, let us revisit, briefly, the first movement pattern taught in Lesson 1. Using your Arch and Flatten pattern as a model, I will guide you in exploring how you might assume initiative in delving more deeply into any of these teachings.

Practice: Lie on your back with your knees bent and your heels drawn up toward your buttocks. Begin to prepare yourself in your mind to inhale as you slowly arch your lower back up from the floor. However, before you start with any movement, pause right at the cusp of the actual movement, and prepare *in your mind only*—that is, just think about doing your Arch and Flatten as if you were suspended halfway between the thinking and the actual doing. Notice, how even at the thinking or planning stage, prior to actually implementing any deliberate movement, there are a whole host of action dynamics occurring throughout your body. Notice how much undirected (heretofore unconscious) movement occurs throughout your body at this movement preparation stage. Observe, for example, how your lungs prepare to breathe in anticipation of matching breath with movement. Feel the ever-so-subtle shift in the arch of your back and the equally subtle press into your heels, and let those feelings guide you in sensing the muscular nuances that precipitate them. These sensory awarenesses and others may be new for you, but the subtle shifts themselves are ever present. Noticing these aspects—aspects otherwise relegated to your unconscious and automatic realm—represents a major advance in gaining enhanced self-sensing and self-control.

Just at this threshold—during your motor planning phase—is where you can indulge yourself fully at the very brink of separation between action and stillness, between substantiality and insubstantiality, between doing and not-doing. It is here that your "in"tention alchemizes into action, and where your "at"tention offers the greatest prospects in terms of enhanced sensory motor awareness and control. At this brink, you become best able to intervene consciously in restoring unconscious and habitual muscle patterns to a level of full and healthy function. The choice is yours to make, at any time and at any point during your somatic visitations, to decelerate fully into the moment and explore at this boundary.

CHAPTER 14

FUNCTIONAL DIFFERENTIATION OF YOUR LUMBAR, THORACIC, AND CERVICAL SPINE

The following transcript, a condensed excerpt from a second movement pattern developed by the author, is designed to help you in further differentiating the movements of your spine and waist. As with the patterns taught in Chapter 13, you may prefer to have another person read these directions aloud as you follow along. You may also find it helpful to acquire an expanded prerecorded CD version of this lesson series; see Resources section. Please review the Cautionary Note at the beginning of Part 4 before proceeding.

An oft heard complaint from older folks, meaning those of middle age or older, is that their spine no longer affords them quite the same degree of freedom and rotational flexibility as it did when they were younger. Nowhere is this decreased rotational flexibility more apparent, or more annoying, than when you need to turn your head for pulling out into traffic or for looking behind while driving your car in reverse (perhaps you have some other pet peeve about this limitation). As a teenager you probably simply whipped your head around to see your way clear when backing up your car, never giving the turning of your body or the twisting of your neck a second thought. Now, however, if you're over forty or fifty years of age, you've probably started to notice some decline in this flexibility, as well as a nagging sense of nostalgia for youthful pliability.

Your spine has three degrees of rotation—forward/backward, tilting from side to side, and twisting or spiraling. Your spine provides the primary framework (along with the ribs that attach to your thoracic vertebrae) for the most central components of your motor system, namely the large muscles of your back, abdomen, and trunk. Therefore, the freedom and flexibility with which you are able to rotate, flex, and tilt your spine underscores your body's freedom and flexibility overall. Looseness and flexibility must start from your core, and stem from there outward.

The lessons that follow are designed to guide you in exploring the first two of these three degrees of motion, and in learning how to differentiate their function to increase the level of command you exercise over your body. Lesson 1 addresses spinal torsion, enabling you to gain, maintain, and more precisely control your ability to twist your spine and look around behind (useful, as noted, for backing up your car, among other tasks). Lesson 2 addresses forward/backward movement aspects, enabling you to more fully arch and extend your back to the rear and flex forward.

For either of these lessons, you may find practicing before a full-length mirror to be helpful. Though a mirror is not necessary to your practice, the visual feedback afforded by a mirror can offer a more objective perspective, allowing you to see your posture and note for improvements, and to compare for discrepancies in sidedness as you go along. The exercises that follow are taught from an upright standing posture, but you may also try adapting them to sitting in a chair,[1] or even while sitting on the floor. For best results keep all movements slow and methodical with an eye to process over goal.

Note: "Pause and practice" indicates that you pause after a set of directions and allow yourself time to practice a pattern (usually three to five repetitions or so, though lingering is encouraged), before advancing on. Take your time and do not rush through or force any movements if you wish to gain best results. Move, at all times, according to your own ability and within your own comfort range.

---

1 Note: if practicing from a chair, be sure your chair is sturdy enough to provide a safe and secure base.

Lesson 1, Part 1

Practice. Start by standing upright with your feet positioned at about shoulder width. A full-length mirror, if available, will be helpful in providing ongoing feedback as this lesson unfolds. Keep your feet firmly rooted in place and casually, and without momentum, begin turning your body around from side to side as if you were looking to the rear. Perform these movements without any agenda other than to notice what the movement feels like. Pause and practice. As you turn to your full limit at either side, make note of some reference point (ideally determined by wherever your nose is pointing) so that you can measure as you go along for improvement in your range of motion.

As you continue with your side-to-side turning, notice if you tend to initiate the movement from your lower spine (which includes your waist for purposes of this work), or from your upper spine (meaning your head and neck), first in turning, and then in returning. That is, does your waist turn first, and then your middle back and head follow its lead? Or do you lead with your head and then pull the rest of your spine around to follow? Explore this closely. Pause and practice.

In the interest of differentiation, try reversing the order of whichever part you lead with. If you usually lead with your head, try leading with your waist, or vice versa. Notice if reversing your natural tendency feels easy or if it requires a concerted effort on your part. Notice also if this adjustment has any effect on your range of motion. Pause and practice.

Reflections. Your spine is divided into three sections, lower (lumbar), middle (thoracic), and upper (cervical) [Figure 14-1]. Each of these sections is engineered to move freely according to the design of its respective vertebrae and according to variations in disc structure. Five vertebrae make up your lumbar section;[2] twelve vertebrae comprise your thoracic spine (your ribs attach to these), and seven vertebrae make up your neck, or cervical spine. It is

---

2   There are also five fused vertebrae that form the sacrum, plus the coccyx, or tailbone, housed within the sacroiliac.

partly the ratio of disc thickness (discs being the spongy cushions between the vertebrae) to the height of the individual vertebral bodies that determines the full potential range of movement between any two vertebrae.

Your greatest potential for spinal movement according to all possible planes occurs in the cervical spine, followed by the lumbar, and then the thoracic spine.[3] Your actual individual functional range (as opposed to the maximum human potential range) is influenced as well by supporting ligaments and, of course, by the ability of your muscles to comply with motor signals sent from the brain. Your more encompassing multidirectional mobility aside, movement that is rotational only (twisting from side to side) is greatest at the cervical spine, somewhat less extensive at the thoracic spine, and quite restricted in the lumbar spine.[4] Discounting the mechanical limits of your spinal components, any tightness and habituation occurring in the back, shoulder, or neck muscles, caused by sensorimotor amnesia, will reduce your range of motion accordingly.

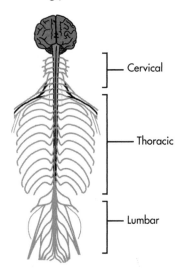

Cervical

Thoracic

Lumbar

Figure 14-1.

---

3 Kapandji, *The Physiology of the Joints.*
4 Kapandji stipulates potential axial rotation to either side as slightly more than ninety degrees, though less than ninety degrees is normal.

One common complaint as people age is that the cushioning discs between the vertebrae atrophy. This is a major contributing factor to people shrinking from the full stature of their youth as they grow older. I submit that this atrophy can be abetted, if not caused outright, by the archeology of insults discussed in earlier chapters. I believe chronic stiffness (habituation) in the large muscles of the back, as well as in the smaller para-vertebral muscles, can be implicated in exacerbating disc degeneration.[5] It is a well-known fact that bones develop according to the stressors (or the absence thereof)[6] to which they are submitted. It seems only common sense, therefore, that the stress of chronically tight muscles in your back can cause or contribute to spinal degeneration. However, if you can prevent or eliminate the chronic stress that characterizes sensorimotor amnesia to maintain a fuller voluntary control of your back muscles, your back will stay healthier and feel younger and more flexible even as you age. Additionally, you will be less prone to the shrinkage that ordinarily accompanies the aging process. The purpose of the exercises in this section is to accomplish just that, by improving your ability to differentiate the muscles that control each of the three sections of your back.

Practice. Turn your body again to the right...and then back to center. Turn again, only this time see if you can turn from your lower back only, without any independent movement occurring at your middle or upper spine. Your middle and upper spine should not turn (or fail to turn) to any degree beyond where your waist turns. Repeat this a few times until you are confident that just your lower back/waist is turning. Pause and practice.

Come back to center. From here, turn only your upper spine (head and neck) to the right. Unless you have preexisting issues with your neck, mov-

---

5   This "shrinkage" may also be attributed to calcium depletion from the vertebrae themselves. Given that bones develop in accordance with the stresses placed on them, it's possible that unhealthy muscular stress on the skeletal components can contribute to loss of bone density, as well as degeneration of discs.
6   Susan E. Brown Ph.D., *Better Bones, Better Body*. Keats Publishing, 2006. "Adults... restricted to bed rest... lose almost 1% of their lumbar spine mass per week." Brown notes that astronauts in weightless environments are also subject to rapid bone loss.

ing just the neck as differentiated from the rest of your back should feel easy enough, up to a certain range. Notice if there's a point beyond which the turning of your neck also tends to recruit the turning of your shoulder and middle spine. Keep the turning of your neck just short of that point. Return to center.

From here, things get a bit tricky. Try to maintain your lower and upper spine as perfectly stationary to the front while you attempt to turn only your middle spine to the right. You will probably find it more than a little challenging to differentiate your middle spine as separate from the parts above and below. Nevertheless, give it a few tries (but remember, no straining), making note of where in your body you feel challenged. Pause and practice.

Now rest for a moment with your body recovered to center. Don't be too concerned if attempts at differentiating your middle spine seemed beyond your ability. We'll revisit this maneuver later on.

Your next task will be to try isolating and moving each section of your spine in progression, starting with the lower spine. Calling into play just your lumbar spine, turn as far as you can, without straining, to your right. Hold your lower spine there, and continue turning with just your middle spine to the right. Hold at this juncture and continue turning with just the upper spine, your head and neck. Now unwind yourself. Repeat this sequence a few times until you feel a clear sense of differentiation between your lower, middle, and upper spinal divisions. Pause and practice.

Implementing the same segmented progression—lower, then middle, then upper spine—turn and hold briefly at full turn. From here, recover to the front by unraveling your spine in reverse order, first returning your neck only, until your nose is aligned directly over your navel. From there, re-center your middle back so that your shoulders align squarely over your hips. Finally, bring your waist fully back to center. Practice this, incrementally around and incrementally back, until it starts to feel natural. Pause and practice.

Try reversing your order of movement in another way. Begin by turning just your upper spine to the right. Practice so that you are able to move your neck as distinct from your middle and lower back. As you hold your neck to the right, add in the rotation of your middle back only. While holding your head and middle back to the right, add in the rotation of your lower back. Practice so that you have a sense of being clearly segmented—upper, then middle, then lower spine—in turning your body around to the right. As with your earlier movement, unwind yourself by reversing and recovering incrementally, recovering your lower back and waist to the center first, followed by your middle back, and then your neck. Pause and practice. And rest, taking a few minutes to stroll about as you feel for change in your body's freedom.

Let's add a next level of challenge. Turn your lower back to the right and hold. Add in the turning of your neck only, leaving your middle back temporarily out of the mix. Recover to center. Pause and practice. Now, turn your lower and then upper spine again, and from this position you may add in the turning of your middle spine. Notice if adding in the middle spine last allows for an increased range of motion in rotating around beyond your original reference point. You can even hold with the lower and upper portions already turned and practice articulating just the middle spine as a way to feel how the thoracic spine can be differentiated from the spinal segments above and below. Pause and practice.

It's time to reintroduce one of our earlier movements, the middle spine differentiation that I assured you we would revisit. Starting from your front position, try turning first your lower, and then middle, spine to the right. Pause, and return. Again from your starting position, try turning only your middle spine, followed by your upper spine, to the right. Pause, and return. Moving slowly, try isolating just your middle spine to the right (be gentle and conservative here) as you maintain your waist and your head oriented to the front. As you gain some measure of success at this, you may sense that this articulation has you feeling less tall, as indeed will be the case due to your spine bowing (don't worry; it's not permanent). Do this several times, then rest. This completes Part 1 of Lesson 1 on the right side.

Take a few minutes and stroll easily about, comparing for any differences in how the two sides of your body feel.

At this point you may proceed to reverse the patterns we've covered on the right over to your left. (Note: If the prospect of reversing on your own seems daunting, you may refer back through the previous section and simply substitute right for left, and vice versa, wherever sidedness is indicated.)

Once you have completed all your patterns on both sides, recover to your starting position. With your feet firmly rooted in place, casually and without undue momentum, turn your body around from side to side to compare for overall improvement in the ease and facility with which you are able to rotate your body. Comparing for before-and-after improvements can be helpful at any juncture.

Reflections. Mathematically speaking, there are quite a few possible variations on the incremental turning and re-turning combinations explored above. Feel free to experiment to further enhance your ability to differentiate.

Note: Before experimenting with the new patterns taught next in Part 2, make sure you've accomplished a comfortable command of the patterns taught in Part 1.

In Part 1, I provided detailed instructions for moving your body according to certain patterns, all to the right side, before abandoning you to figure out on your own how to apply those same patterns to your left. I left you to your own devices at reversing the pattern, not because I'm mean, lazy, or negligent, but so you could have the experience of exercising your own brain power in mapping out those patterns in reverse. Reflect back for a moment on how you went about implementing that reversal of patterns for yourself. Was it easy? Or did you find it especially challenging? Did you rely on some strategy, such as the suggested reversing of all the earlier directions for right and left sides, or did you opt to trust your instincts? However you tackled that reversal, I offer you my assurance, right off, that I will not abandon you in similar fashion here in Part 2.

Lesson 1, Part 2

Once you feel adequately in command of the lessons presented up to this point, there is a second component you might care to explore in developing a fuller control of your rotational abilities. It is during this next round of practice that you will find use of a mirror—any mirror—to be most helpful in anchoring your attention forward. Absenting a mirror to hold your own gaze, you can make your best effort to stabilize your head by fixing your gaze at some forward point. And, you will need "twinkle toes."

With your eyes and head held as fixed forward and maintained as steady to avoiding bouncing, begin to implement a series of the tiniest in-place steps to "walk" the whole rest of your body, from your middle spine down, one third of your turning potential to the right. In other words, instead of initiating the turn from the top down with your stance fixed, walk your body around, starting from your feet and working upwards, all the while keeping your head and neck fixed precisely in place. Note: The emphasis on moving according to "your turning potential" implies that you stay well within your safety range and move in subjective, versus objective, "one third" increments. Keep your eyes fixed forward and tiny-step your feet back to center, and then tiny-step one third of your turning potential around to your left, again moving your whole body except for your head and neck. Try this, back and forth, for a few rounds. Pause and practice.

Let's repeat the same pattern, only this time walk your feet around two thirds of your turning potential to the right. And then two thirds of your turning potential back around to the left. You'll probably notice that at some point beyond a one-third shift, your feet keep turning even as your middle spine stabilizes at its limit. Take a few minutes and try this maneuver going in either direction, noticing how this compares to your earlier turning patterns, and also for your overall range of motion.

If and when you feel ready to try going just a little further, you can attempt the same pattern, now walking your feet around until your body is in (for you) a fully rotated position, just as it was earlier when your lower, middle and, upper spinal sections that were leading the move. Remember, though, no straining. At the very least, your friends and family should find this entertaining. Meanwhile, the differentiation of rotating your spine, by starting from your lower body, as opposed to rotating your spine starting from the waist up or from the head down, should provide for some interesting comparisons and afford you yet another way of thinking about how you can organize your body.

Caution: Keep in mind throughout these patterns that the purpose is to gain differentiation and intelligence, i.e., enhanced control of your muscles, and not necessarily to stretch or contort your body. Increases in range of motion as a result of practicing these movement patterns may well ensue, but any increase is best achieved by relinquishing habituated tightness that unnaturally restricts your range of motion. Take care to resist any temptation you might have to coerce your body into stretch mode. Your primary interest here (as with all somatics exercises) is in reversing any net loss in flexibility that you may have incurred, more so than in accomplishing any net gain. Genuine and lasting net gain can only occur after full recovery from net loss.

Lesson 2

Lesson 2 concerns itself with optimizing your ability to flex and extend your spine, forward and backward, along a sagittal plane. This lesson, like Lesson 1, may be practiced standing or sitting (with an added measure of safety, please, if you opt for a chair). Note, however, that a posture other than standing may dictate separate consideration in how you organize your spine according to the directions that follow.

Practice. Begin standing upright in a balanced posture with your feet positioned parallel and about shoulder width apart. Let your arms hang freely by your sides and keep your knees slightly flexed for best stability. Carefully arch your spine and extend your body backward, just enough to explore your range of motion. Note: If your balance is already compromised due to "age" or by a preexisting condition, you may want to keep some support near at hand, such as a chair back or a countertop. Also, if you suffer from back pain, be gingerly in your arching. If you have any doubt about your ability to arch safely, consult with your health advisor first.

Notice as you arch if your tendency is to bend more, or less, from your lower, middle, or upper back, and in what order. Notice, also, where your spinal arch begins and where it ends. Pause and practice.

Next, starting from a neutral upright position, slowly bend your body forward, letting your arms hang toward the floor. Notice for the relative involvement and participation of each of your spinal segments. Pause and practice.

Reflections. While arching your back, you may find it helpful to register some visual reference point overhead or to the rear. In flexing forward, you'll find it helpful to note how far down along your legs or how close toward the floor your hands reach. Both these "before" measurements will serve as frames of reference against which you can measure for any gains you make in improving your forward/backward range of motion.

Reflections. Mathematically and practically, there are fewer possible variations (assuming you are not skilled as a gymnast or contortionist) to experiment with in flexing and extending your spine as compared to the earlier rotational patterns. Even so, the movement patterns that follow may help you to substantially increase your range of motion as you learn to move your spine in a more intelligent and controlled manner. Any tightness or inflexibility you feel due to SMA notwithstanding, the human spine has quite an impressive potential range of forward and backward flexibility, up to 250 degrees in per-

sons who are optimally supple.[7] As you proceed through the following movement patterns keep in mind that safety is paramount, and that any increase
you achieve in range of motion is secondary in importance to accomplishing
an enhanced sense of differentiation along your front/back plane.

Practice. As you prepare to arch backward again ("arching backward" is
actually a bit of a misnomer), focus on just your lower spine. Instead of lean-
ing backward with the upper portion of your body from the lower body, try
to draw just your lumbar vertebrae forward, over the waist, to better sense
the arching in your lower back. Maintain your lumbar arch as safely centered
over your waist, such that if you were observed from a side view you would
appear to be extending your belly forward rather than reaching your upper
body backward [Figures 14-2a & 14-2b]. Pause and practice.

Next, hold as you arch your lumbar section forward...then arch your
mid-spine forward as well. You'll notice that arching your mid-spine forward
will have the additional effect of drawing your scapulae (shoulder blades) in
closer together. Here, as before, observed from the side you would appear to
be extending your ribs forward. Pause and practice.

Next, lift and puff out your chest as you lift your chin and tilt your head
back, lengthening the front of your neck. Throughout, your body should
remain safely balanced over your waist. As you continue to practice these
sequences, turn some of your attention to your breath. Begin with a lower
abdominal breath as you arch the lumbar spine, and allow your breath to
progressively fill and expand the thoracic cavity as you add in each extra bit
of arch. Pause and practice.

Once you are comfortable with the segmented progression into this
arched posture, replete with full breathing, shift your attention to recovering from your arched position in reverse increments, working from the up-

---

7 According to Kapandji, the flexion/extension of the three sections of the spine is as follows:
lumbar at 60°/35°, thoracic at 105°/60°, cervical at 40°/75°.

per spine down. First bring your chin forward until your head is at neutral to the middle spine; then sink your chest, and finally relax your belly back to flat so that you finish standing properly erect. Pay attention to how you progressively release the breath as each section of your spine returns from its extended position forward to neutral. Practice arching back and recovering like this several times.

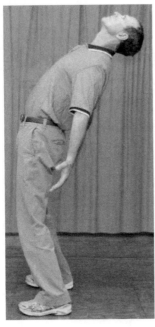

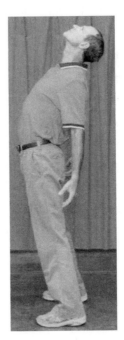

Figure 14-2a. Incorrect, body is overarched.

Figure 14-2b. Correct, body is safely centered.

Next, let's experiment with a forward bending, or flexing, version. Begin by allowing yourself to droop forward with your arms hanging to the front. Notice where your hands hang in proximity to the floor and make a mental note of this for future reference. Recover back up to neutral, being sure to rely on bent knees in bringing yourself erect. Practice drooping forward again, taking special note of how your spine flexes. Does it move smoothly, akin to the action of a roll top desk, or is it more inclined to move stiffly, in starts and stops, like a series of rusty hinges? Pause and practice.

Working from the top down, allow just your head to flex forward, and notice how the muscles at the base of your neck and upper shoulders (just where the upper and middle segments of your spine meet in juncture) prevent the neck from folding forward beyond a certain range. At this juncture, sink your upper chest—hollowing it as if your chest were a sail billowing inward from the wind—and observe how this sinking of your chest frees your head and neck to droop more fully forward, your chin narrowing the gap to your chest. Notice also how sinking your chest inward has the reciprocal effect of bowing your middle spine back to the rear. Practice this several times, gently and gradually increasing the involvement of your middle spine, so that with each forward flex you allow your middle spine to bow a little more toward the rear. In recovering from each flexion keep in mind that it is safer, in terms of spinal mechanics, for you to invoke a roll-top-desk-type recovery than to try lifting from your middle spine as if it were a rigid unit.

In the next phase of flexion exhale and fold forward, as before, until you sense yourself at just that juncture where your thoracic spine meets your lumbar spine. From this juncture, exhale some more and progressively draw in your belly. Feel how this rounds the thoracic spine, helping your abdomen make way for your body to continue flexing forward and down. Notice where your hands dangle in comparison to your earlier reference point. Can you observe any improvement? You may note that in addition to being an excellent means of increasing your ability for spinal flexion, these maneuvers are also effective in lengthening tight hamstring muscles. During recovery from this forward position be sure to keep your knees slightly flexed to minimize any strain on your lower back.

When recovering from your bent forward position take care to lift first from your lumbar, then from your middle spine, and finally from your neck, unfolding again in the manner of a roll top desk. Remain conscious of the role of your breath in facilitating these progressions throughout. Pause and practice.

Variations. It bears mention that these arching and flexing maneuvers along a sagittal plane can also be practiced from different starting postures, for example from a forward kneeling posture, or even lying down on either side (which markedly changes the effects of gravity as a variable), as a way to further enhance your capacity for spinal differentiation. Feel free to experiment once you feel comfortable with the basic patterns.

Reflections. Because this is an exercise designed to help you recover differentiated movement, versus one designed to stretch, strengthen, or condition your body, a mere several slow repetitions in any given practice session should be adequate to the task. There is no need to push your body to, or even near, its limits to effectively stimulate the sensorimotor pathways that govern these movements. Regular short and focused practices will prove more effective than protracted sessions. These movement patterns appear, outwardly, as short and simplistic, yet they can be profoundly effective, providing you practice according to a somatic mindset, i.e, slowly and methodically, with your attention set to process over goal.

During forward and backward flexion and extension move slowly and consciously at all times to avoid any inadvertent reliance on momentum. Always pay close attention to how your body might try to "compensate," e.g., shifting weight more onto either leg, to keep balanced during any deviation from your front/back plumb line. During these movement patterns you can enhance the beneficial effect by actively employing your breath, not just its fullness, but its placement as well, to keep your body safe while exploring for your natural range of motion.

This concludes Lesson 2.

Reflections. This completes this excerpted lesson series in differentiating the movements of your lumbar, thoracic, and cervical spines. During any given round of movement practice you must take care to set genuinely conservative limits for yourself in neither over-reaching nor over-practicing. Keep in mind also during practice to always move methodically and with an exploratory mindset for best and safest results. Try to move as if you were discovering these abilities for the first time each and every time you practice. Remember, the primary purpose of this work is to improve your muscular intelligence through differentiated movement. Any gains you achieve in flexibility or range of motion are simply icing on the cake.

CHAPTER 15

SWIMMING IN ALL DIRECTIONS
TO FREE YOUR SHOULDERS

The following patterns can be practiced from a sitting or a standing position. However, unless there is a compelling reason to sit, I recommend standing because this will allow you to experience your full potential for integrating the movements of your elbows and scapulae (shoulder blades) with the whole rest of your body. As with all other somatics patterns, the suitability of the described movements hinges on the absence of any contraindication to practicing them safely. Please review the Cautionary Note at the beginning of Part 4 before getting started, and consult with your doctor or somatic educator before practicing the following patterns if you have any doubt.

As with the previous patterns taught in this section, you may prefer to have someone else read these directions aloud as you follow along. An expanded version of this lesson series is available in prerecorded CD format, see Resources in Chapter 17.

This pattern series stemmed from my abiding interest in Tajiquan. As a Tai Chi teacher I am regularly challenged to impart the nuances of Tai Chi to students who arrive for studies with bodies that may be already burdened by the effects of sensorimotor amnesia. Nowhere are the dissonant effects of SMA more likely to evidence themselves than in imbalanced and tight shoulders. Given the prominent role of the hands and arms in Tai Chi, as well as the importance of relaxing the upper body for a low center of balance, this is a matter of some concern as constriction in the shoulders and upper back effectively precludes the correct expression of Tai Chi's embodied principles.

During Tai Chi classes, I often guide my students in somatics patterns to address these same concerns. However, whereas most somatics patterns are practiced while lying down, I sought to develop a movement series for freeing tight shoulders that could be seamlessly integrated into a martial arts warm-up routine while in a standing posture. The following is just such a pattern. Aside from being suitable for martial artists, the shoulder patterns that follow will prove invaluable to golfers, swimmers, tennis players, and other sports and fitness enthusiasts.

Part 1

Begin by positioning your hands as interlaced behind your head. Arrange your flexed elbows positioned somewhat to the front, so that you can easily see each elbow from its own sided eye, i.e., right eye sees right elbow, etc.

Practice. Starting at your right, begin moving your elbow in a small counterclockwise pattern, as if you were tracing with your elbow tip to draw a smooth circle just two–three inches diameter. Pause and practice. After several slow repetitions, gradually enlarge your circling pattern to five–six inches. Pause and practice. Next, try enlarging your elbow circle to the size of a dinner plate (again, staying within your ability). Pause and practice. Finally, if your range of motion allows, begin to expand your movement so that your upper arm and elbow resemble a forward swimming stroke—up, over and out, down, and back—the only difference being that you still have your right hand interlaced with your left hand behind your head. Pause and practice. Stop, release, and rest your right arm.

Reflection. While performing the described movement pattern, divide your attention so that you're dually aware of the circle that you're tracing with your elbow and of any involvement occurring at your arm's scapular (shoulder blade) connection in back. The larger your circle in front, the more likely you'll notice the role of your scapula, either in its freedom to move freely with the elbow or, conversely, as a hindrance to the elbow's smooth circularity.

Go ahead and repeat this pattern, step by step, on your left side, moving your elbow now in a clockwise, versus counterclockwise, direction so that your overall movement still has you moving in a swimming forward direction. Refer to the steps above if you need a reminder.

Once you've completed these patterns on the left side, try combining the two sides into an alternating pattern, using both right and left elbow circles. Start with small circles and gradually enlarge until both arms are moving smoothly as if you were swimming in the air with an overhand stroke. The larger you make your circles, the more likely it is that other parts of your body, including your torso and waist, will become involved in some way as part of the overall movement. As the scope of your circling motions expand, try to be especially sensitive for any "stickiness" that might indicate sensorimotor amnesia. If you feel stickiness, resist the urge to speed up or to plow through the resistant area. The goal here is not to circle your arm at any cost, but to use these patterns to identify and relinquish such SMA as may be revealed. Throughout, keep your head upright and forward facing, but avoid strain. This will be easier to accomplish if you let your hands slide and glide freely behind your head and neck. Pause and practice.

Variation. Having started with small elbow circles that gradually evolved into larger circles which also recruited the scapula to move circularly, try reversing the order of progression. See if you can begin by circling just the scapula, that is let the movement emanate from the scapula, with a minimum of elbow rotation. Try this with either shoulder in turn before combining the two sides. Pause and practice.

Rest both arms down and stroll about. Let your arms swing freely. Notice how your shoulders feel as you gently shrug them this way and that.

Part 2

Movement. Begin with your arms and hands positioned as in Part 1. This time begin circling your right elbow in a small clockwise (opposite) direction. Continue, adhering to the same model of progressively larger circles established in Part 1. Instead of swimming forward, though, you'll be swimming in the manner of a backstroke. Practice just on your right side, experimenting with incrementally larger circles, before reversing over to the left.

Reflection. While practicing the same patterns on your left, notice how each side compares to the other in all regards, including range of motion, ease and fluidity of movement, and the level of concentration required to articulate your movement. Notice, also, how the reverse direction compares overall to the original direction of movement. Is forward or backward circling easier, freer, or more expansive?

Movement. Try combining both arms so that you truly do look as if you are swimming backward. Remember to let your interlaced hands glide freely behind your head. Throughout, it will remain essential if you want to achieve full and lasting benefit that you move attentively according to the precepts laid out earlier in this book. I might sound like a broken record, but I can't emphasize strongly enough that it will be your mindful attention to your movement, as much as the movement patterns themselves, that facilitates enhanced freedom of motion and a feeling of fuller voluntary muscular control.

Once you've finished this pattern, rest and stroll about.

Make sure that you indulge yourself some practice time on the movement patterns covered thus far, enough so that you're comfortable with all aspects, before advancing on to Part 3.

Part 3

Movement. Start by positioning your hands again interlaced behind your head. Move your right elbow counterclockwise just as you did in Part 1. Come to a halt after a few basic circles. Move your left elbow also in a counterclockwise direction for a few circles. Stop briefly...and resume, moving both elbows in counterclockwise unison.

Reflection. Your elbows will be circling in the same direction—in tandem like two bicycle wheels traveling from right to left. Both scapulae will be turning counterclockwise, exactly opposite (asymmetric) from one side to the other. Notice how this feels. Stop and rest briefly before reversing direction. When you feel ready you can try "bicycling" your elbows left to right in a clockwise direction. Rest your arms and walk about, feeling for any newfound freedom in the swing of your arms and shoulders.

Part 4

Movement. Your next round of patterns will be characterized by movements that are symmetrical (as opposed to alternating). Start with your hands again interlaced behind your head, and move both elbows slowly forward...then down...then back...and then up...in perfect symmetry, each elbow moving as a mirror image of the other. Your right elbow will be circling counterclockwise while your left elbow circles clockwise. As your elbow circles become larger your arm movements will increasingly resemble the butterfly stroke of a swimmer.

Reflection. Notice if the supposed mirror imagery of your moves is perfect or if it appears distorted. You may find yourself challenged in your best efforts to maintain a symmetrical circularity, especially as your circles enlarge. Remember, don't try to force a larger range of motion. Instead, pay attention to where in your body you may be feeling resistance and restrictions to your movement and focus your attention there. Rather than force your way through resistance, try to listen for any resistance "non-confrontationally," so your resistant areas can gradually release on their own terms rather than being disarmed coercively. The best way to engender this kind of cooperation from your body is to keep your movements slow and deliberate. Stop and rest your shoulders.

Movement. When you feel ready, you can resume with your elbows circling in the opposite direction as if you were working slowly up to a double-arm overhead backstroke. As with our previous models, start small and expand from there. Also remember to move slowly (Did I say that already?). It's not unusual for movement patterns such as these to be accompanied by some degree of "crunchiness," which can seem disconcerting at first. Keeping your movements slow and deliberate, versus momentum based, will minimize crunchiness and help you to avoid strain. Once you've achieved your own comfortable limit, and before fatigue sets in, stop and rest.

Reflection. With both of these double-arm forward and backward patterns you're likely to notice more of a tendency for your spine to undulate as your movements expand. In noticing this tendency, you might try experimenting to see how you can exploit the natural undulations of your body to advantage to augment the rotational potential of your arms and shoulders.

Part 5

For your final movement patterns, let's dispense for the time being with circles and try something a little more linear. Position your hands as interlaced behind your head and your elbows pointed out to either side. Organize elbows and shoulders so that you have a straight alignment from one elbow across through shoulders and body to the other elbow. Try to maintain this alignment as you reach, just a little bit at first, with the right elbow to the right. Then relax and reverse with the left elbow reaching out to the left. Alternate, gradually extending your reach to the side with either elbow to involve increasingly more of your shoulder and body in the movement.

Reflection. Notice how freely your scapulae glide as separate from the back as either elbow extends out to its side. Notice also how your body organizes itself by shifting hips and weightedness to maintain balance.

Try performing the following one time in either direction. Starting with your hands and elbows aligned as above, try reaching out again with your right elbow and shifting all your weight to the right, "fixing" your body there. Hold your body in this position as you shift only your elbows and scapulae across to the other side, so that the rest of your body (and its weightedness) is moving exactly opposite from elbows and shoulders. Then reverse. Now relax.

Once you complete your practice session, allow your arms to hang freely while you walk about. Notice the newfound freedom in your upper body, in general, and the easy swing of your arms, in particular. This completes this lesson series.

End note. Feel free to experiment as regards the specific plane in space of your elbows during any of the covered patterns.

CHAPTER 16

WHERE BREATH MEETS QI:
PERINEAL BREATHING

GET YOUR QI UNSTUCK
AND IMPROVE YOUR LIBIDO

Please review the Cautionary Note at the beginning of Part 4 before proceeding.

Readers may find the patterns that follow to be useful in several regards. First, in keeping with the theme of our somatic overview, the following exercises may result in a renewed or enhanced sensory awareness in the muscles and nerves of the urogenital region, this due both to the relinquishment of chronic tension (SMA) in the surrounding musculature and to an increase in your ability to differentiate the perineal region. Accompanying this renewed sensitivity, it is quite possible that you may (over time and with continued practice) experience some increase in libido as these subtle movement patterns allow for an increase in the flow of both blood and Qi to area tissues that may have previously suffered from blood and Qi deprivation.[1] Problems typically associated, directly or indirectly, with compromised blood or Qi flow to

---

1 Thus far I have only made passing references to "energetic" concerns and considerations, as these generally fall under the purview of TCM. However, this particular pattern series calls for some mention of Qi due to the possibility of concomitant energetic effects. If you are not inclined to consider the flow of energy via the acupuncture meridians, feel free to disregard these references.

the urogenital region include impotence, diarrhea, prostatitis, incontinence and frequent urination, hemorrhoids, menstrual and menopausal difficulties, constipation, and more.

In seeming contrast to what I noted earlier in the Q&A section, regarding there being substantive differences between somatics and Taijiquan, this chapter offers a hybrid movement pattern. These movements are based on somatics principles as they can be applied to certain physiologic components I learned in a qigong context long before I'd even heard of somatics. I practiced these movements as adjunct to a more encompassing Taoist energy practice for several decades. Seeing great value in the adjunct movements themselves, I have conscripted and refashioned them according to a new (somatics) agenda. In keeping with Hanna's more global philosophy, nearly any movement can be experienced somatically if practiced in the correct manner.

Dr. Thomas Hanna's brainchild was conceived not only as a practical methodology such as has been expounded throughout this book, but as a philosophy for living in and through the body in the most intelligent and organized way. Pioneer though he was, Tom Hanna was neither the first nor the last insightful person to orchestrate movement patterns designed with the goal of better living in one's body through self-sensing. Other disciplines as well, and according to varying agendas, have sought to recruit the body's compliance toward this end. Some methods have encouraged self-sensing for its own sake. Others have cultivated self-sensing as the means to another end. In the section that follows I guide you in practicing a series of (often exceedingly subtle) moves that will likely challenge your ability to control your body at a level of nuance. Rest assured, you CAN learn and accomplish this chapter's subject matter if only you persist in a patient and process-oriented fashion. The rewards you gain over the long term will make your efforts worthwhile.

As with the guided patterns in earlier chapters, you may prefer to have another person read these directions aloud as you follow along. A prerecorded (and much expanded) version of these lessons is also available in CD format; see Resources.

Perineal Breathing

Conscious and deliberate breathing into the depths of your abdomen on a regular basis offers a range of valuable benefits. Such breathing has the effect of exercising and toning both the thoracic and urogenital diaphragms.[2] From the perspective of TCM, this approach to breathing also stimulates the body's Wei Qi function to keep your internal Qi pressure strong. This, in turn, strengthens and supports your immune system and flushes blood and Qi through the lower abdominal area, which can be helpful in preventing or alleviating lower back pain and sexual energy problems respectively. Finally, by toning the lower abdominal area, you will be less susceptible to the depleting effects of energy leakage, ala TCM, via the sexual and eliminative orifices.

In the sections that follow, I introduce a series of breathing exercises designed to help you build up your skill toward perineal proficiency. I recommend that you take the time to grasp each level of skill thoroughly before proceeding to the next level. Individual abilities may vary, but for newer practitioners it is generally advisable to think in terms of weeks or months to gain proficiency, versus hours or days.

Part 1

This level entails simple abdominal breathing, not altogether different from what you might encounter in any yoga or martial arts class. To begin, sit or stand upright with your hands folded comfortably over your abdomen just below your belly button. Breathe through your nostrils and use the intention of your mind to guide and follow your breath down into the lower abdomen, just behind and slightly below the navel (known in TCM as the Dantien), so that your abdomen fills and expands outward on each in-breath. Then, allow

---

2 The urogenital diaphragm, aka pelvic floor or pelvic diaphragm, is a muscular partition composed of muscle fibers, i.e. the levatores ani and the pubococcygeus, including the parietal pelvic fascia on their upper and lower aspects, as well as associated connective tissues which occur in the lower pelvis. The pelvic floor separates the pelvic cavity above from the perineum below.

your abdomen to relax and flatten inward on each out-breath. Breathe slowly and deliberately at first. Practice in rounds of three, six, or nine consecutive breaths and repeat at your own discretion.

Part 2

Next we advance to even lower abdominal breathing, first, and add in what I call small sip breathing.

2-A. Shift the focus of your attention from your navel area downward to just behind the pubic bone (known as the Lower Dantien).[3] Begin by breathing as in Part 1, only with your breath aimed even lower. You might find it helpful, at first, to place a hand over the pubic bone to help anchor your attention there. Repeat three, six, or nine breaths as in Part 1. Most people find this lower belly breathing to be moderately more challenging than breathing to the naval area. A few rounds of practice sessions should suffice to familiarize yourself with this technique so that it begins to feel comfortable.

2-B. You will now learn small sip breathing. Under normal circumstances when you breathe your inhalation/exhalation cycle proceeds linearly. That is to say, you take one breath in for each breath out, and so on. Small sip breathing entails a departure from this pattern. Here, you will take a series of in-breaths without releasing your breath out. In order to do so without straining (very important!), it will be necessary for you to precisely regulate each inhalation so that you take in only a small amount of air with each in-breath. Each of your mini-inhalations will still be directed into your lower abdomen, as before; but in this round you'll make each in-breath deliberately a bit "terser" as it inflates your pubic area. You might liken this to puffing short bursts of breath into a balloon as opposed to exhaling one long breath—only

---

3   The pubic bone, aka pubic symphysis, can be felt just deep to the surface, at the midline, as a bony protuberance above the genitals.

here you will be sipping your breath in, instead of exhaling it out. Remember to inhale through your nostrils.

If you lack previous experience at breathing disciplines, I recommend you begin with a moderate goal of three–six sipping inhalations before releasing your breath. Try this several times, at least, before advancing to any higher number of repetitions, up to a maximum of nine or eighteen inhalations. In the context of the qigong method I alluded to earlier, practitioners often strove for more than one hundred consecutive intakes of breath without exhaling, and even at that without straining! Now perhaps you can appreciate why this method is called the "small sipping" breath and not the "big sucking wind" breath. In any case, as our agenda here is quite different from that original qigong context. I recommend fewer and more precise breaths for greater gain. With a little practice, you can experiment with up to eighteen breaths, being careful not to overdo it. As you might imagine, you'll become able to regulate your breath to a very fine degree as you improve your skill at this practice.

Did I mention the importance of not straining when practicing your sipping breath? Particularly, be careful to confine your intake of breath to just the lower abdominal area as it is important to avoid creating any tightness or constriction in your chest area. Your personal progress at this method won't be measured according to how fast you increase the number of breaths, or by the speed or vigor with which you breathe during practice. Instead, pay attention for the subtler nuances of controlling and targeting your breath as a finely tuned mechanism. As you familiarize yourself with this method, try to rely increasingly more on the intention of your mind and increasingly less on your body's mechanical force in guiding your breath. In other words, try to think it, or *will* it, without forcing it.

Part 3

Now you are ready to shift the focus of your attention, as well as your breath, all the way into your perineum.

Anatomically, your perineum is that small area just behind the genitals and forward of the anus [Figure 16-1a]. However, for the purposes of this work, we will take a little license, ala TCM, and regard the perineum as extending from just behind the genitals fully back to the coccyx [Figure 16-1b]. When you first attempt to breathe into your perineum, you'll find it helpful (assuming you're not in mixed company) to use the tips of your fingers to press in just behind the genitals. This will help you to anchor your attention at the perineum and receive immediate and tangible feedback on the effectiveness of your breathing technique. Just as your naval and lower abdomen inflated palpably with the in-breaths you practiced earlier, so will the perineum respond to a correct in-breath. It would be awkward, to say the least, to observe your own perineum visually. By using your fingertips to press up against the perineum you should be able to feel your perineum pulsing gently downward as you target your breath down into it.

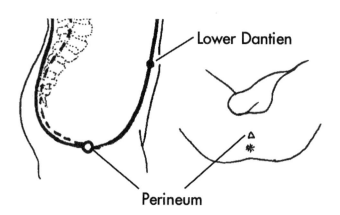

Figure 16-1a. The anatomical perineum.

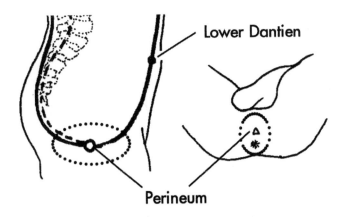

Figure.16-1b. "Expanded" perineum (dotted circle).

3-A. Begin by breathing into your perineum in much the same manner as you did into the naval and lower abdomen. Draw in one breath, followed by a soft release out. Practice this until you are comfortable with it. This style of breathing will likely be quite a bit more challenging even than the lower abdominal breathing of the previous exercise. Try not to become frustrated if at first you fail to experience the desired results. This may take a bit of practice.

3-B. Once you feel yourself able to breathe into the perineum so that it inflates palpably downward, you can advance to sipping. As with the previous exercise, you can inhale a series of short sipping breaths, three, six, nine, and so on, into the perineum, optionally relying on your fingertips to gauge your body's response to each breath. Remember, don't strain.

3-C. Your previous maneuvers were the easy part (sorry). Next, you will divide the perineum into at least three, and optionally five, distinct sections: front, middle, back, and optionally, left and right [Figure 16-2]. In the sections that follow you will learn how to breathe into each of these sectors as separate and distinct parts of a whole. Please refer to Figure 16-2, as indicated.

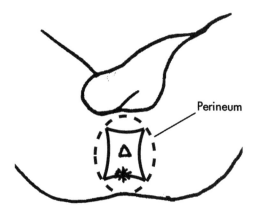

Figure 16-2. The five sectors of the perineum.

First, focus on the front, or forward, part of your perineum. Use your mind to direct your breath to that just area immediately behind the genitals, but forward of the anus (see area in dotted circle, just above the rectangle). Use a shorter in-breath, rather than a deep inhalation, and pull up (pucker) the perineum slightly, enough so to just barely tense, but not clench, the pubococcygeal (PC) muscles[4] as you draw in your breath. Release the breath along with any effort from your PC muscles. Repeat this pattern until you can coordinate the breath and the tensing and release of same comfortably.

3-D. Move your attention to the middle of the perineum, at the anus (lower center of rectangle). As you breathe to this middle sector, just barely tense or pucker your anal sphincter muscle, being careful to avoid any tensing at the front part of the perineum. It may take a good bit of practice before you're able to effectively differentiate between these two target areas. Release both the breath and your sphincter muscle. Practice this skill until you are comfortable with it.

---

4   For men, activation of the pubococcygeal muscles will also recruit the cremaster muscle that pulls up the testes.

3-E. Next, advance your attention to the back (rearmost) part of your perineum, behind the anus and just beneath the coccyx (area in dotted circle, just below the rectangle). When you breathe to this sector, your breath should be accompanied by a very slight tensing or puckering of the muscles just below the coccyx. If you do this correctly, you should also feel a very slight outward tilting, or tugging, of your tailbone. Here again, be careful to not involve the front or middle parts of the perineum. When you release the breath, relax your coccygeal area completely, and your tailbone will relax back down.

3-F. If (and once) you feel ready to include the right and left sides of the perineum into your practice, you may proceed as follows. The directions are the same for both sides so I will guide you for the left side only, and you can adjust accordingly for the right side. Bring your attention to the middle area, at the anus. Sip and pull up once, then release. Shift your attention from center to just left of center. Try to keep the middle sector relaxed while you direct your breath to the left side of your anus. This should be accompanied by a barely perceptible tensing of the anal sphincter on the left side only. Release and relax as before. Practice this several times on the left side before practicing on the right side.

3-G. Once you feel competent at breathing into and articulating each individual section of the perineum you can begin to orchestrate a more sequential practice pattern, as follows: Inhale and hold a single small sip at the front, then a sip to the middle, then to the back, and then to the left and right sides of the perineum in turn, for a total of five sips, before releasing the breath. Pause and practice this.

Once this feels comfortable you can try adding, and holding, a second sip to each target area before moving to the next point, for a total of ten consecutive sips. Eventually, if you feel ready, you can triple your sips, for a total of fifteen small sipping breaths before exhalation. Remember, no straining—just inhaling with an increasingly precise and nuanced puckering of the associated musculature. At this point it should become evident why we spent so much time and effort earlier learning the small sip skill.

Once you've achieved a relative command of this method you ought to be able to condense an entire practice session into as little as five or ten minutes, or somewhat longer if you prefer.

Both during and after learning the methods taught in this chapter, once you are ready to conclude any given practice session (in which you are not proceeding on to a next section), I recommend you repeat a few rounds of your simple Abdominal Breathing, as covered in Part 1, to bring closure to your practice. This concludes the practical guidance for Perineal Breathing.

Please keep in mind that a convenient feature of these breathing practices is that you can resort to them almost anytime and anyplace. Whether you are standing in line at the supermarket or riding the bus to work, you can always discreetly practice your abdominal or perineal breathing skills. With practice, you'll find yourself able to rely increasingly on just your attention and intention in guiding the breath into the abdomen or perineum, and also in differentiating the muscle minutia of these areas for the proscribed benefits. Enjoy.

Remember, also, that there is an impressive array of long-established movement patterns that were designed by Thomas Hanna Ph.D. I heartily recommend these. See Resources in the next chapter for further information on these media items.

CHAPTER 17

FINAL WORDS

I am a firm believer in the potential of somatics to meet the health and wellness needs of a broad spectrum of individuals and, by extension, to ease the burden on at least one aspect of a growing national healthcare crisis. I've covered many bases: athletic injuries, kids, martial arts, sex, those who are old and decrepit, folks who are breathing challenged, accident and injury victims, and those who don't have a choice about growing old but sure don't want to become decrepit. This list offers but a sampling of those who stand to benefit from the HSE method.

Somatics is self-directed healthcare—a means of personal sustainability—for the average person. This is something you can do, and you can do it for yourself, and even by yourself. Somatics can put you more in charge of your own life.

All of what I've written in this book is offered in service to mankind, in belief, as Thomas Hanna was quoted early on as saying, "...to see enough change happening to say...I've helped things along a bit...It has to do with loving other people and being concerned with the human condition."...and with helping others become free in their bodies in the truest sense of the word."

I want to close with one more sentiment left with us by Hanna, "As we grow older, our bodies—and our lives—should continue to improve, right up until the very end. I believe that all of us, in our hearts, feel that is how life should really be lived." I trust you agree, and I hope that what I've shared herein makes a positive difference in your life.

Resources—Where to Go from Here

Now that you've familiarized yourself with somatics and the many possibilities it holds for you, where do you go from here? That depends on what your own personal agenda entails. If your body is in pain or out of balance, or if you feel your body ravaged by the effects of sensorimotor amnesia due to a lifetime of living and an archeology of insults, you are probably excited at the prospect of finally being able to do something about it. You can start by seeking out for a qualified somatic educator in your area.

Important note: To avoid confusion, readers should be aware that there are two separate somatics brands, so to speak, each offering its own best interpretation of the late Thomas Hanna's work. At the Novato Institute in California, interested persons can find Hanna Somatic Education®. At the Somatic Systems Institute in Massachusetts one will find Prime Somatic Education®, aka clinical somatics. These teaching facilities offer different brands of somatics, but their approaches are fundamentally similar, each adhering according to its own best understanding to the principles and methods laid out by Thomas Hanna. All of what I've written in this book applies regardless of whether you opt for "Hanna" somatics or "Prime" somatics. In either case your most important consideration will be your choice of an individual educator best suited to your needs.

If you don't already have a practitioner in mind there are several helpful resources I can recommend. Readers are welcome to learn more about somatic education and related products by visiting my own website; www.painandmobility.com. You may also direct inquiries to:

Association for Hanna Somatic Education, Inc.
P.O. Box 2484, Napa, CA, 94558-0248.
Phone/fax 877-766-2473
www.hannasomatics.com

On this website you'll find a wealth of resources, products, and information, plus a roster of certified somatic educators, listed according to geographical location. For other helpful sources for information, practitioner referrals, and products:

Somatic Systems Institute in Northampton, MA.
(where I received my training)
877-766-2746
www.somatics.org

Novato Institute in Novato, CA. (the original)
415-897-0336
www.somaticsed.com

If you are intrigued and want to follow up with somatics simply as a way to achieve and maintain better health for yourself and your loved ones, you may prefer to explore somatic movement patterns on your own. You can learn these patterns directly from a certified educator, many of whom offer dedicated classes in movement patterns as separate from their clinical practice. These teachings are also available in listening formats[1] on electronic media, and are a wonderfully effective way to gain many of the benefits of somatic at your leisure and in the comfort and convenience of your own home. Most of these guided series contain six–eight individual half-hour(-ish) lessons. They are easy to follow and sufficiently intriguing that you'll find yourself wanting to listen and follow along over and over. There is an extensive selection of lesson themes available, focusing on different physical conditions or areas of the body. Many are guided by Thomas Hanna personally. Others are offered by somatic educators who have followed in Hanna's footsteps. I offer a collection of guided patterns of my own composition, available on my website. Other

---

1 Our position as somatic educators is that improving sensorial awareness is most effectively facilitated by guided audio narration, versus visual media.

selections and formats can be found at some of the URLs listed above.

Finally, if you find yourself so enthused as to be interested in professional training for a career in somatics, information on training programs can be found at the websites mentioned above. Both the Novato Institute and the Somatic Systems Institute offer training programs for practitioner candidates. The programs are well designed and very professional. Somatic education is a fast-growing field offering a whole new range of wellness possibilities to a population in need. As of this writing there are fewer than two hundred practitioners worldwide who are certified in the methods developed by Thomas Hanna. This number is increasing rapidly as training programs expand and more people become aware of the efficacy of somatic education and opt for careers in this growing field.

LEARNING MEDIA

BY THOMAS HANNA

AUDIO: Somatic Exercises[TM] narrated by Thomas Hanna

The Myth of Aging: Somatic Exercises to Control Neuromuscular Stress
Somatic Exercises: The Complete Cat Stretch
Somatic Exercises for the Legs and Hip Joints
Somatic Exercises for the Hands, Wrists, Elbows and Shoulders
Somatic Exercises for the Neck, Jaw and Skull
Somatic Exercises for the Lower Back
Somatic Exercises: Freeing the Whole Body from Center to Periphery
Somatic Exercises for Delicate Backs
Somatic Exercises for Full Breathing
Somatic Exercises for Feet, Knees and Pelvis
Somatic Exercises for Rounded Shoulders and Depressed Chests
Somatic Exercises for Protruding Bellies
Somatic Kinesiology

Other Publications and Media by John Loupos
BOOKS
Inside Tai Chi: Hints, Tips, Training & Process for Students and Teachers
Exploring Tai Chi: Contemporary Views on an Ancient Art
Tai Chi Connections: Advancing Your Tai Chi Experience

DVD

Tai Chi Connections

CDs

Movements for Sensing & Freeing the Sacrum & Cranium (2006)

Functional Differentiation of the Lumbar, Thoracic, & Cervical Spine (2009)

Swimming in the All Directions to Free Your Shoulders (2009)

Where Breath Meets Qi: Perineal Breathing & More: Get Your Qi Unstuck &

Improve your Libido (2009)

Swaying in the Breeze: for Improved Balance & Proprioception (2009)

To order:

Visit www.painandmobility.com

or contact:

John Loupos

130 King St., Cohasset, MA 02025

781-383-6822

SUGGESTED READING

Baars, Bernard J. *In the Theater of Consciousness: The Workplace of the Mind.* New York: Oxford University Press, 1997.

Begley, Sharon. *Train Your Mind Change Your Brain: How a New Science Reveals Our Extraordinary Potential to Transform Ourselves.* New York: Ballantine Books, 2007.

Brown, Ph.D., Susan E. *Better Bones, Better Body.* New Canaan, CT: Keats Publishing, 2006.

Cozolino, Louis. *The Neuroscience of Psychotherapy: Building and Rebuilding the Human Brain.* New York: W.W. Norton & Co., 2002.

Crossman, Alan R. and David Neary, M.D. *Neuroanatomy*, 2nd Ed. Edinburgh: Churchill Livingstone, 2000.

Doidge, M.D., Norman. *The Brain That Changes Itself: Stories of Personal Triumph from the Frontiers of Brain Science.* New York: Viking, 2007.

Garoutte, Bill. *Survey of Functional Neuroanatomy*, Greenbrae, CA: Jones Medical Publishing. 1981.

Gladwell, Malcolm. *Outliers, the Story of Success.* New York: Little Brown, 2008.

Goldberg, Elkhonon. *The Executive Brain: Frontal Lobes and the Civilized Mind*. Oxford: Oxford University Press, 2001.

Goleman, Daniel. *Social Intelligence: The New Science of Human Relationships*. New York: Bantom, 2006.

Hamill, Joseph and Kathleen M Knutzen. *Biomechanical Basis of Human Movement*. Hong Kong: Lippincott, Williams & Wilkins, 2006

Hanna, Thomas. *Somatics*. New York: Addison-Wesley Publishing Co., Inc, 1988.

————, *The Body of Life: Creating New Pathways for Sensory Awareness and Fluid Movement*. Rochester, VT: Healing Arts Press, 1979.

Hesson, James. *Weight Training for Life*, Pacific Grove, CA: Brooks Cole Pub, 2006.

James, William. *The Principles of Psychology*, Vol 1. New York: Cosimo Classics, 2007.

Juhan, Dean. *Job's Body: A Handbook for Bodywork*. Barrytown, NY: Barrytown/Station Hill, 2003.

Kapandji, I.A. *The Physiology of the Joints*, Vol. 3, Edinburgh: Churchill Livingston, 2004.

Knaster, Mirka. "A Somatic Approach to Yoga." *East/West*, 1989.

Lacher, Denise B., Todd Nichols, and Joanne C. May. *Connecting with Kids through Stories*. London: Jessica Kingsley Pub, 2005.

SUGGESTED READING

Metzinger, Thomas. *The Ego Tunnel: The Science of the Mind and the Myth of the Self.* New York: Basic Books, 2009.

Pollan, Michael. *In Defense of Food: An Eater's Manifesto.* New York: Penguin Press, 2008.

Ramachandran, V.S. *Phantoms in the Brain: Probing the Mysteries of the Human Mind.* New York: Quill, 1998.

———. *A Brief Tour of Human Consciousness.* New York: Pi Press, 2004.

Ratey, M.D., John R., *Spark: The Revolutionary New Science of Exercise and the Brain.* New York: Little Brown, 2008.

Rock, David. *Your Brain at Work.* New York: Harper Collins, 2009.

Schwartz, M.D., Jeffery M., and Sharon Begley. *The Mind and the Brain, Neuroplasticity and the Power of Mental Force.* New York: ReganBooks, 2002.

Siegal, Daniel. *The Mindful Therapist.* New York: Norton, 2010.

Szpunar, Karl K. and Kathleen B. McDermott, Ph.D. *Cerebrum: Emerging Ideas in Brain Science, 2008.* Washington, DC: Dana Press, 2008.

Victoroff, Jeff, M.D. *Saving Your Brain: The Revolutionary Plan to Boost Brain Power, Improve Memory, and Protect Yourself against Aging and Alzheimer's.* New York: Bantom Books, 2002.

Weil, Andrew, M.D. *Spontaneous Healing.* New York: Ballentine Books, 1995.

————. *Healthy Aging: A Lifelong Guide to Your Physical and Spiritual Well-Being*. New York: Knopf, 2005.

Werner, Ruth. *A Massage Therapist's Guide to Pathology*, 3rd Ed. Hong Kong: Lippincott, Williams, & Wilkins, 2005.

GLOSSARY

Afferent (sensory) nerves: The nerves that deliver information *to* the central nervous system and brain.

Brain maps: Specific processing areas in the brain delegated for specific tasks or functions.

Cerebral cortex: The layer of gray matter on the surface of the cerebral hemisphere that is responsible for intellectual faculties and higher mental functions, as well as coordinating sensory and motor information.

Default setting: In the brain/CNS, this represents the baseline tonus for a muscle while in its supposed resting state, when it is not being deliberately recruited for an action.

Dendrite: Short and branched extensions of the nerve cell body that receive and integrate signals coming from the axons of other neurons, and convey the resulting signal to the body of the cell.

Green Light reflex: Ala Thomas Hanna, a chronic engagement of muscles associated with the body's "let's go" response, usually involving the large extensor muscles of the back of the body.

Efferent (motor) nerves: Neurons that activate muscle cells.

Habituation: A state in which a muscle retains some degree of chronic contraction, or stuckness, even when the brain is not actively calling it into play, usually due to a disruption in the afferent/efferent neural feedback loop. Not to be confused with stimulus habituation, aka desensitization in Classical Conditioning.

Kyphosis: An exaggerated convex curvature of the upper back/neck, i.e., humpback.

Landau reflex: This describes the activation of the body's dorsal extensor (back and neck arching) muscles, with typical onset around four or five months of age.

Long-term (synaptic) potentiation (LTP), aka LTSP: The means by which repeated firings between two neurons at a synaptic junction results in that process becoming more efficient.

Lordosis: An exaggerated concave curvature of the lower back.

Mirror neurons: These neurons are understood to activate both on their own and in response to another person being observed performing a same behavior.

Momentum: A property of dynamic force that keeps objects (or dispositions) moving in a same direction, unless and until overcome by resistance.

Neuroplasticity: The brain's ability to adjust its circuitry according to changing circumstances.

Neuron: A type of cell that receives and sends messages, often from the body to the brain, or vice versa.

Occipital ridge: The base of the skull at the back of the head where the cranium meets the neck.

Proprioception: The process by which specialized nerve sensors strategically located throughout the body provide continuous feedback to the brain about bodily position.

Protocol: In somatic talk, this (generally) is any one of three prearranged sequences of methods and techniques designed to address Red Light, Green Light, or Trauma issues.

Qigong (aka Chi Kung): A generic term that describes a field of energy-based disciplines generally stemming from traditional Chinese martial, spiritual, or healing disciplines. Qigong can be categorized as medical, alchemical, or simple. Most Qigong practices fall into the latter category.

Reciprocal inhibition: The deliberate tensing of muscles to stimulate a relaxation response in their antagonist (opposite) muscles.

Red Light reflex: Ala Thomas Hanna, the body's chronic activation of muscles associated with the fear or apprehension response, aka startle response, usually involving the large flexor muscles of the front of the body.

Reflex pattern: A pattern of habituation learned by the body due to some conditioning stimuli.

Sacrum: The large triangular bone at the base the spine, housed within the pelvic "bucket." It is comprised of five fused vertebrae and the coccyx, or tailbone.

Scapulae: The wing-like shoulder blades located at the upper back, comprising part of the shoulder girdle.

Sensorimotor amnesia (SMA): A state in which all or part of the brain's ability to sense the behavior of a voluntary muscle has been compromised due to a disruption in the afferent/efferent neuromuscular feedback loop.

Stretch reflex: Aka the myotatic or segmental reflex, the reflexive contraction of a muscle, instigated by intrafusal muscle fibers, when that muscle and its attached tendon have been pulled or stimulated by rapid, violent, or excessive stretching.

Subcortex: The lower and more primitive region of the brain below the cerebral cortex.

Taijiquan (aka Taiji/Tai Chi Chuan/or Tai Chi): An ancient form of Chinese martial arts, characterized by slow movement practice, and premised on the acquisition of certain intrinsic principles.

Trauma reflex: Ala Thomas Hanna, the tendency of the body to enter into an habituated protective or compensatory (splinted) posture, often in response to real or perceived danger or injury, and generally characterized by asymmetry.

Wei Qi: An immune system component, i.e, the body's first line of energetic defense, ala TCM, against illness and injury.

INDEX

ABOUT THE AUTHOR

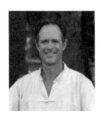 **JOHN LOUPOS, M.S.,** is a certified Hanna (and Certified Clinical) somatic educator. He serves on the board of directors for the Association for Hanna Somatic Education, Inc. and maintains a private clinical practice in Cohasset, Massachusetts.

John Loupos has practiced and taught martial arts since 1966. His martial arts background includes Okinawan Karate, several styles of Chinese Kung Fu, Taijiquan, Liu He Ba Fa, Bagua, Hsing-I, qigong, and more. John also has a background in Classical Homeopathy. He conducts seminars nationally on martial arts and on somatics.

The author welcomes reader comments and questions.

jadeforest@comcast.com

www.painandmobility.com